Charmaine Grace Brown

GRACE,
THE GIRL WITH CELLS THAT WERE
SICKLED

How It All Started

GRACE, THE GIRL WITH CELLS THAT WERE SICKLED
Copyright © 2025 by Charmaine Grace Brown

The content of this publication is based on actual events. Names may have been changed to protect individual privacy.

This material is not intended as a substitution for medical advice. Please consult a physician before undertaking any changes to diet, exercise, or medication.

Softcover ISBN: 978-1-4866-2536-9
Hardcover ISBN: 978-1-4866-2404-1
eBook ISBN: 978-1-4866-2537-6

Word Alive Press
119 De Baets Street Winnipeg, MB R2J 3R9
www.wordalivepress.ca

WORD ALIVE
—PRESS—

Cataloguing in Publication information can be obtained from Library and Archives Canada.

I DEDICATE THIS book to my mother, Ruthlyn Shaw-Cunningham, for caring with support, prayers, and encouragement—a mother who never gave up through the horrific times.

To my siblings, nieces, nephews, and friends who were there to assist with whatever I needed.

To Ohma and Alfred, who were there physically carrying me.

And to the greatest of all, God, for showing up when it was least expected.

CONTENTS

ACKNOWLEDGMENTS

BRAVO TO THE healthcare workers who effortlessly help in compassion and gentleness when caring for those in need. Those who advocate for and follow up with their patients wherever they are located or relocated. The ones who stop other healthcare providers from mistreating the vulnerable. You are acknowledged and appreciated.

GRACE, THE GIRL with Cells that were Sickled is a series of true stories that include educational elements. It is about the life of Grace, who has been living with sickle cell disease (SCD) for over fifty years.

Grace experienced challenges, support, associated illnesses, debilitating ulcers, healing, decision-making, and both negative and positive mental health changes. The hospital admissions, discharges, insults, and family socialization aided the hope for wellness.

The lack of research on the disease in the initial phase of her diagnosis led to dissatisfaction with wound care, pain management, and adequate mental health. Grace had to adjust in many ways, but it was troublesome trying different treatments.

Navigating through the school system with bullies and defending herself led to anxiety and fear. The dreams, brokenness, desires to be healed, and hate she had toward God all led to disastrous behaviours.

She had planned to hurt herself when God stepped in to claim her life. Do you think she received healing? Do you think God loved and forgave her for the hate she had toward him?

HOW IT ALL STARTED

Greatness and obscurity fluctuate on a continuum.

GRACE WAS BEAUTIFUL with flawless olive-coloured skin. It glowed in the sunlight like soft silk. Her eyes were big and brown with yellowish sclera; they sparkled when she laughed. Her face was small and could be held in the palm of her tiny hand. There were no visible eyebrows— just bare skin where her eyebrows should be. Her eyelashes were fine and scattered and gave no shade to her eyes.

She had a flat-bridged nose that perspired when she was hot and tired. She had small ears and medium-sized lips. Grace's yellowish-white teeth were scattered in her mouth, especially in the bottom gums. Her hair was black, with fine strands—soft in the hands, wool-like, and short on top of her head. She had small ears and a long straight neck.

Grace seemed underweight but played a lot, so her weight was adequate for her activities. She had five brothers and one sister whom she loved. Her sister Darlene was taller, and as beautiful as she, and her brothers were handsome.

Rose, Grace's mother, had seven children: Nick, Andie, Dean, Darlene, Grace, Mick, and Jim. Only Darlene, Mick, Grace, and Jim enjoyed spending time together. They went all out with games, assignments, teasing, or relaxing. Mick and Darlene protected Grace at all costs because she was frail, and her meager stature caused them to fear that grass straws (as they were called in Jamaica) would break her tiny feet. Andie was bossy and played tricks on them. He took the money they sometimes got from their dad, Lester.

Andie bossed them around to do chores and always requested they stay inside the house doing assignments or reading. He required them to be cleaned and fed. He did not socialize with other people, especially the tenants, although they lived in a tenement house.

Grace hated it when Andie was around because he was too strict and boring. He always told them to bathe, sleep, read, or be quiet. The children had Monday to Friday after school and Saturdays until 6:45 pm to play without a person of authority around. Grace and her siblings were unruly when Andie was not around.

After Rose and Lester separated, Rose took Grace and her family to live in a big old rackety house that seemed to be made from red dirt, mall powder, and other building materials. The house was torn down in places and had peeled walls. It was a tenement building with seven bedrooms, three kitchen areas, one bathroom, an outhouse, and outside bathing areas.

There was old rusty zinc on the roof. Some places leaked when it rained. It had a massive yard with red dirt, trees, grass, and herbs, and there were cultivated fields that the kids roamed for pleasure. The house had two entrances, one from the road in front and the other from the side. There were a lot of trees and shrubberies surrounding the outskirts of the house.

The house was about five hundred metres from both sections of the main roads. It was on a big plot of land that was covered with weeds and surrounded by broken-down perimeter walls. There were two big round tanks made of stone and cement. One was at the back of the house and was used for garbage; it had a tall pear tree in the middle that occasionally bore fruit. The other was at the side of the house. Gutters attached to the house channelled rainwater into it for domestic purposes. When it had water, the tenants were happy because they did not have to search for water on other people's properties. The tank was about twelve feet deep, eight feet in diameter, and two feet wide. This allowed people to access the water and still prevented a person from falling in.

There was another tank that sat on four iron columns, up in the air between the other two. This tank was made from concrete. After a rainfall, it contained water that was not safe to drink. This tank also contained Tika Tika River fish. As dangerous as these tanks were, the children included them as play areas. They had no sense of danger.

Grace sat in the big tenement yard on the red dirt, which was hard and slippery, especially when it rained. She focused on Jim while waiting for one of her siblings to relieve her. She needed a chance to play. On weekdays, when school was in session, Grace focused on Jim, who was twelve years younger than her.

Each child took turns babysitting Jim, who occasionally played in the big yard. The children knew they would be in trouble if any-thing should happen to him. Their bodies were covered in red dirt as they played. Grace's teeth were red and mucky from eating the dirt. She loved the taste of it, especially the hard pieces that were difficult to chew.

Grace tried to hide her secret habit, but her teeth were the evidence. They sat at the side of the house and played jacks and balls, as well as Chinese skip, hopscotch, hide-and-seek, and any other games that came to mind. There was screaming, laughing, and calling each other thieves when they were unsatisfied with their winnings.

They snuck through their bedroom windows when no one was watching, ran through the fields, climbed trees, bounced elastic bands against the wall, and tried to win each opponent's pawns. Their play time was endless: marbles, books, and cards. They used old tires to make cars; carton boxes for trucks; and oranges, limes, or bottle corks for wheels.

These children were able to make games out of anything. Sometimes the games were vicious and exhausting. They would run around in the rain, slide in the mud, and try to swim in puddles of water. Grace and her siblings played barefoot, which made it easier to get around without slipping and falling. They did not know better. It was natural because of the warmth outside all the time. They lived in a small town called May Day in Mandeville, Manchester, Jamaica. Running around in shoes could have caused sprained ankles and broken bones. Bare feet provided more stability and safety for their continuous playtimes.

Grace and her siblings were creative, unique, and thoughtful extraverts; they were unbelievably skilled at seeing everything as a game. They were always outdoors when Andie wasn't home. The children helped Rose with tasks in her restaurant and ran errands, like going to the abattoir to buy meat.

They were carefree and childish. Grace hated losing and was competitive, but so were the tenants' children and her siblings, especially Mick. When she lost a game, especially Ludo, she cried in sadness and shame, but the more she cried, the more they teased her. One tenant, Miss Dory, would encourage her not to cry but to be more charitable when the others won. She tried over and over but lost again and again and sobbed to the point of snivelling.

Grace was a happy child but afraid of breaking her bones from falling, so she was careful when she played outdoors. She never knew what it meant to be in need. People around them provided for their well-being. They protected Grace from rain, excess heat, fatigue, hunger, and bullying. She, Jim, Mick, and Darlene were a gang. They ate, slept, laughed, cried, and entertained themselves. And they were mischievous. This gang was thicker than thieves. Dean, Andie, and Nick were usually with friends or working to earn money.

Darlene, Grace, and Mick took turns caring for Jim, who was a baby. The school they attended worked on a shift model where the morning shift ran from 7:15 am to 12:00 noon, and the evening shift was from 12:15 to 5:00 pm. These children were brilliant in school and were top students.

Grace and Mick were on the morning shift, and Dean and Darlene were on the evenings. Jim was Grace and Mick's responsibility at the end of the morning shift and Darlene and Dean's responsibility at around 6:00 pm, but most times, Dean was unavailable. He stayed with a crew of boys and made friends.

Jim was loved by all and was a happy, chubby baby. Grace and her siblings' duties were to watch, feed, bathe, and keep Jim safe until Rose was home. Andie, Dean, Darlene, Grace, Mick, and Jim all lived with Rose, a single parent. Nick lived with another family. Rose hired two sitters, one for the morning and the other for the night. The sitters were inexperienced with active children who were full of energy. The sitters were shy and didn't know how to manage these little tricksters. These middle-aged female helpers needed the funds, so they took the job. They neglected their chores, except cooking and protecting the youngsters from harm.

There was no set schedule, and these children had no examples to follow. Andie or one of the tenants assisted them in attending school on time. If given the opportunity, Grace and her siblings would play day and night. There was no concept of time.

The school was problematic at times. When they arrived at school, everyone was already in class; this was when they realized they were late. They were flagged for being late by the homeroom teachers under a big oak tree. Students lined up under this tree. The line would run past the school gate and about a thousand metres toward the main road, filled with students waiting to be whipped.

Going to school was hectic for Grace because her little hands meant her hygienic needs were poorly met. At times, she smelled of urine, which she could not identify but was teased about by other students. Grace would wet the bed regularly, not from laziness but because she could not control her bladder at night.

Occasionally, Rose placed plastic on the mattress, with linen, to help the mattress from getting wet with urine. There were odd times when her mother would wake her and assist her to the washroom. Those were successful nights that Grace was happy and proud about. Andie helped by encouraging her to wash her body properly.

Rose ensured that all uniforms, clothing, and linens were washed and pressed. Hair was braided neatly, assignments completed, school bags cleaned, and contents of writing pads, outdated textbooks, and pencils were prepared on Sundays. The children needed newer study guides, but Grace's mother seemed clueless about the significance of up-to-date textbooks. They would have contributed to better grades, although Grace and her siblings still got excellent marks.

Grace was never punished at home. The flogging only took place at school. She was unable to get accustomed to this horrifying act yet could not escape such punishment. She was so young and did not know how to explain to her teacher that her lateness was unintentional. She was so scared of being flogged that, sometimes at night when she thought about it, her bed-wetting got worse.

She did her best to leave on time. When she ran to school, she was breathless and felt faint. The walking was also tiring and caused her heart to pound in her chest. If they'd had a responsible adult to guide them in their schooling or explain things to their teachers, it would have prevented the floggings.

When Grace was twelve years old, as she and her siblings played in the big yard and the cultivated fields, she noticed she had been limping for several days. When she walked, the pain got worse. Grace realized something was wrong because it was difficult for her to run and play the way she frequently did.

Grace was too young to understand what the issue was. She was having pain in her right lower leg at her inner ankle. A small spot there hurt underneath the skin. The area was darker than her usual skin tone—painful, fluid-filled, and odd-looking.

Running through the field toward the bamboo trees caused excruciating pain. She sat at the corner of the house on the slope near the tank and cried softly. With her wet brown eyes, Grace took the opportunity to watch Jim while her siblings roamed the open fields and climbed the bamboo trees to the end of their chutes.

Silently, Grace watched her siblings and the neighbour's kids climb to the end of each chute. Their weight brought the whole bamboo shaft to the ground. This was fun for them as an outdoor sport. They laughed in excitement and Grace desired to be part of the play.

This made her feel alone, although Jim was beside her. He seemed to understand that Grace was not feeling well. He was clinging to her, hugging and kissing her wet, tear-stained face, cooing all the while.

Each day was more fearful than the last because the pain in Grace's right ankle got worse. The fluid-filled area spread like wildfire and contained a small hole that leaked foul-smelling drainage. This blister-like area started peeling off and leaving exposed flesh that was dreadfully painful.

Grace, her siblings, and the tenants looked at her leg and wondered what was happening. Her mother was not there; if she had been, then maybe a doctor would have been out of the question. Rose was so busy, and making time to assess that inner ankle could be disastrous for the family finances. Her mother's absence from the workplace had to be planned. It was difficult for Rose because she had to provide adequately for her children.

The fluid-filled, malodorous, blackened, and swollen area opened wider and became an ulcer. The outer area was red and tender, and the sore hurt with every step she took. Grace's functionality declined significantly due to the severe pain and open wound.

About six months after the right inner ankle started, the same thing occurred on the left foot. It was insufferable to have two wounds with the same magnitude of pain. No one knew how to remedy the situation. The doctors were unable to diagnose the problem, so pain management and proper treatment seemed impossible.

Grace's brothers and sister were never sick. She was the only one to be admitted to the hospital in the first nine years of life. At birth, she'd been diagnosed with sickle cell disease (SCD). None of the medical professionals they saw knew the real issues and complications of this disease. They were incapable of educating Rose about the disease or how to keep Grace safe. No one prepared Rose for how Grace's health would be substantially impacted. The realities of this disease were left to everyone's imagination. The name of the disease was intriguing, since none of them knew what a cell was or how it could become sickled.

Grace's family members were only able to repeat the words *sickle cell* to themselves. When people asked about Grace's feet they would repeat these words. Rose did not know how to protect Grace from having a sickle cell crisis (SCC). None of them had any idea how damaging it would be or the extent to which these cells were sickled. It was a term that later became their nightmare, ghost, and tormentor.

Each family member had a story to claim, relate, and fear. Each one regretted hearing or learning about the disease but appreciated what it meant in their lives. It was where Grace realized the viciousness and heart-wrenching effect of such an unusual disease and how it led to severe calamity and destruction all around her.

As Andie guarded his brothers and sisters, he ensured they ate, bathed, slept, and did assignments until Rose was around to take guardianship. Grace's siblings and mother tried to provide physical and emotional comfort for her.

The medical doctors were helpless in providing comfort measures because the medications had not been studied or made accessible to assist her screaming body and aching soul. This was how it all started—how the family learned from trials and errors. How they analyzed, assessed, problem-solved, researched, sought assistance, and taught others about her condition and treatment goals.

This was how it all started and where Grace's life would change forever.

DOS AND DO NOTS

INFORMATION TO PARENTS

1. Observe the changes that your child is experiencing and assess whether they are contributed by illness, anxiety, depression, or other factors.
2. Support your child, especially when they are not doing well. Get better pain management and supportive care when necessary.
3. Speak with other parents or research the problem your child struggles with.
4. Children cannot explain their circumstances, so find other ways—like using toys and puppets—to enhance their communication skills.
5. Seek assistance from nurses, social workers, psychotherapists, doctors, and other supportive people who are available.
6. When children are distracted, it does not mean they are not in pain. Monitor their pain levels and use adjunction therapy like heat packs, blankets, and teas for children who are twelve years or older. Seek assistance from your pediatrician for infants.
7. Advocate for your children because they need a strong voice to protect them.

INFORMATION FOR CHILDREN

1. Tell your parents or guardians if you are not feeling well. Do not be afraid, shy, or ashamed. Remember, you did not cause the issue.
2. Children's pain is underreported and unrecognized (Trottier et al. 2022). Tell someone about your pain, so proper pain management can be administered.

3. Use reading, writing, singing, television, and playing to help you achieve comfort when you are in pain, especially after taking your pain medication and waiting for it to work.

4. Take lots of time to rest and be comfortable. Use toys, pillows, blankets, and your favourite comfort device to assist. Whatever makes you comfortable, if it is a healthy practice, do it. Be comfortable.

THE DOCTORS' VISITS

Arrogance hurts people and puts others to shame unnecessarily.
Arrogance stems from pride, injustice, and inequality.

GRACE WAS COUGHING and had pain all over her body during the night. She slept on Rose's bed comfortably, on the side of Rose's leg. In the morning, Grace did not feel better, so Rose decided to take her to the hospital for treatment. Rose realized that if Grace did not get speedy care, the pain would get worse, and she needed to avoid this at all costs.

The visits to the doctors were ferocious and time-consuming. Rose got ready early because it was a first come, first served hospital. She needed to get back to her restaurant to make money. The drive from their home to the taxi stand near the hospital was approximately three and a half kilometres.

Rose held Grace's seven-year-old hand and guided her. They walked the streets, weaving in and out of traffic and crossing streetlights safely but hurriedly. When Rose reached one of the famous patty shops, she bought them beef patties and orange juice. She always tried to give Grace healthy foods. This meal was conducive to a successful day because the wait at the doctors' clinic could be extremely long.

Grace was tired, but Rose had a time frame to meet and was a fast walker. Grace lingered behind because she was breathless and not feeling well. Rose tried to slow down but did not realize how fast she walked. Grace's heart played high and low rhythms like a drum in her chest. She caught her breath by opening her mouth.

Grace was exhausted but loved to spend time with Rose despite the situation. She was proud of her mom. She loved her and was pleased to be her child. It took about forty minutes to walk from the taxi stand to the hospital.

When they arrived, Rose found a seat for Grace on one of the benches. She went to the registration window and the lady behind the counter, dressed like a nurse, found Grace's chart. The woman looked at Rose through the window that separated them. She whispered something to the lady dressed in plain clothes beside her, then came closer to the window and spoke disrespectfully to Rose.

"You were here two weeks ago with Grace, so why are you back so soon?" she asked with a disdained look.

Before Rose could answer, she continued. "You do not know how to take care of your child. Maybe you should take better care of her instead of coming to the hospital every time."

Her voice was condescending, rude, and harsh. Rose hung her head in shame and tried to get a word in, but the nurse ignored her and told her to sit, as if she were disciplining a child.

Rose called Grace and sat at the benches in the far corner. She turned her head to the wall because people in the waiting area looked at her suspiciously. She hung her head in guilt and embarrassment. Grace saw tears on Rose's cheek and knew her mother was crying because of how the nurse spoke to her. She never cried for anyone to see but did so in private.

Grace felt sad to see Rose crying and inched closer; with a frown on her face, she held her mother's hand. She felt hate in her heart for the nurse. She wished there was something she could do to comfort Rose. At that moment, Grace decided she wanted to become a nurse. She would never treat anyone like that. She would prevent other nurses from talking to patients and families in a derogatory manner. Grace wished Rose knew that she planned to make things better when she got older.

They moved in a queue on benches as they waited to see the doctor. Each time, Rose had to provide stool samples from Grace. There was blood taken. Grace feared needles, so the blood-taking vampires would comfort her while they drew her blood. She was weighed, and her height was measured. The doctor checked her head, eyes, ears, nose, and mouth. He put the stethoscope on her chest and felt her belly. Sometimes her belly hurt under her right ribs. Information was written on a huge chart, and Rose got a note for medications, which she picked up at another window where people waited in line. Rose took Grace to the restaurant after the visit and asked one of the sitters to take her home.

These were the things the doctors did for Grace to help her feel better. The visits occurred at least once a month, unless Grace felt sick in between. Sometimes she would be admitted, and her elder siblings would visit. She spent at least five to fourteen days in hospital on each admission before going home to her family.

DOS AND DO NOTS
INFORMATION FOR PARENTS

1. Do not let anyone degrade you and don't feel ashamed of how you live. Always stand up for yourself.
2. Do not talk down to others because you have a difference in power. Show respect and compassion. Remember, people are doing their best with what they have.
3. Make time for your loved ones, especially when they are not feeling well.
4. As parents, your children love you, and you might be their hero. Do not overlook their admiration in the midst of your busy life.
5. Some people seem like they are doing everything wrong. Do not judge them; instead, uplift them and support their journey. Help them to do right.

6. Some individuals have dreams and aspirations from a young age. Encourage and motivate these desires.

7. Parents, remember that whatever children see, they retain that information because they are sensitive. Do not contradict their knowledge.

8. Stop conceptualizing people's reality. Instead, listen and learn the truth.

BULLYING

Jealousy causes opposition in the world, transforming good to bad, beautiful to ugly, joy to pain, and friend to enemy.

GRACE AND HER siblings attended school daily except for sick days. On days when she was in too much pain and unable to walk, she was left alone with Jim. As a baby, Jim was sensitive to changes around him. He knew Grace was not doing well and tried to cheer her up with baby talk and actions.

When the pain was torturous, Grace had a difficult time getting to the washroom. She limped, but it was agonizing. Out of fear, she sat for a long time, afraid to walk on her feet. Grace wished she could use diapers, but it might be more work. Sick days meant she sobbed, screamed, read, played, rested, and hoped for better days.

At school, she was competitive. At the end of the school year, she got A's. The distance from school to home was about 4.2 kilometres. As short as the distance was, Grace found it harrowing when she walked. She tried to distract herself with her friends or vivid imagination, but moving from one place to another was painful.

Some of her friends from Basic School (Kindergarten) became mean. They called her degrading names, while others laughed. They pulled at her clothes and whispered things to each other. Grace was unhappy when she was teased. She felt discouraged and sorrowful when they called her debasing names. She did not understand what the teasing or angry threats were about.

What happened when one of her friends became her foe? Grace remembered they were together in one class, but after she got first place in fourth grade and jumped to the sixth grade, the problem seemed to start. Her friends were left in a lower grade. One of them was a tall, lanky girl named Judiath. She was angry and acted envious toward Grace. She pulled Grace's hair and pushed her into some bushes at the side of the road. One of the plants, named cowhage, or Mucuna Pruriens, had pods that grew all around in the bushes during warm weather. It contacted Grace's skin and caused severe itching and skin irritation immediately.

At times, when Grace walked alone to school, she feared these girls because she was unable to defend herself, especially with the painful ulcers. It caused Grace to be unbalanced. Sometimes she felt weak and achy.

One day, when Grace was walking to school, the kids planned to fight her at the end of the shift. Grace was scared and did not know what to do. Her bigger brother and sister were on the evening shift and could not protect her. During class, she was worried and lacked concentration.

Grace decided to stay at school until all the students left. This meant that no one would be there to care for Jim, so her siblings would have to be late for their first class, or one of the tenants would have to watch him while he sat in the yard.

Grace sat in a corner on the school grounds after class. She sharpened her pencils and did her assignments while she waited for all the students on her shift to vacate the compound. When all seemed well and the school grounds were emptied, Grace got up and headed to the gate.

On her way home, Grace had to pass Judiath's gate. Judiath lived across from the school's playing field. Grace hid under one of the big trees in the schoolyard and peeped out to see if Judiath was waiting for her in the shadows. She saw no one and started walking toward the road for home, her hands in her uniform pockets while tightly holding her school bag. When Grace reached the road, she ran straight home as fast as a hare. She felt her heart beating like a drum in her chest. She felt faint with throbbing pain in her feet, but she was safe.

Grace's siblings must have passed her while she waited on the school grounds because Jim sat in the big yard when she arrived home. She picked him up and went inside the house. Grace loved her baby brother and hugged and kissed his face tenderly while one-year-old Jim laughed.

She changed, attended to Jim's diaper, and then got dinner for them both. Grace loved being at home because it was safe and away from the problems at school. The dangers lay in travelling back and forth to school, using the school's toilets, and going to the school pipes for water. These places increased the opportunities to be persecuted and became bait for Judiath and her friends.

Grace's sense of normalcy was ripped away due to her wounds and pain. She had no protector and greatly feared the students who taunted her viciously. She sat with Jim in the kitchen for a while before going into the bedroom for a nap. The tenants' children were outside doing chores, and she could not think outside.

Her brother Mick was near the zinced pigpen as he fed Rose's pigs. Grace was too troubled to talk with Mick. After the nap, she took Jim to the back steps so they could play together. Grace played with the set of jacks and balls, rubbing her legs to ease the discomfort. It would be a while before her siblings returned from school. Mick came into the house to put the pig food pan under the sink in the kitchen. She was three years older than Mick, but he was more mischievous. He often misguided the tenants' kids and gave them hot scotch bonnet peppers to eat as cherries or played roughly with them. This would make them cry and feel sad.

The tenants were upset with Mick at times. They shouted and screamed at him to leave their children alone. Mick ran away and made ugly faces at them. This made them angrier. They reported Mick many times to Rose, who slapped Mick and gave him chores that kept him busy.

It was getting dark. Grace and her brothers went to the bedroom to wait for their older siblings. When they were all together, the problems seemed to diminish through their laughter, games, and storytelling. They bathed, but their cleanliness was not the best. The sitters were inadequate and did not assist in their care.

Grace and her siblings needed responsible adults to offer care and protection. They needed assistance with proper hygiene, mouth care, and grooming. Because they were all so close in age, they couldn't help each other properly. The tenants could see that the young children didn't properly understand self-care, so they assisted them when they could. Their mother was pressured to be financially stable so that she could supply their basic needs. Rose trusted the nannies to be competent.

Grace, Mick, and Darlene worked hard. They carried clean drinking water from the pipes at the crossroads, pipes installed by the government. There were times when there was no water in them. When this occurred, the siblings accompanied other tenants in search of clean running water from neighbours' pipes or tanks.

Grace, Mick, and Darlene cleaned, washed dishes, swept, and mopped the house every day, including weekends. They cooked meals and helped each other with anything and everything. Chores were easy for them because they made games of everything they did.

Occasionally, Rose prepared breakfast in the morning and gave them money to buy lunches at school. When their mom left for work, they knew she would return when everyone was asleep. Rose was the only one who loved and took adequate care of them. She bathed and groomed them, and she cooked their meals.

One day as Grace and Mick headed for school, she tried to catch her friends so she could have some company. But her friends were faster and left her behind. Mick also ran ahead. Grace took her time to reduce the pain she felt. Slowing down also prevented her from experiencing shortness of breath, especially when she went over the hills. She was late, and all the other students were far ahead.

When she cleared the first hill, Grace glanced down the slope and saw no one. Judiath was not there. Her heart was beating faster, and she was scared. She went over another hill and looked toward the school gate. Many students slowly walked into the schoolyard. Grace tried not to be late. She didn't want to catch up with some of the students because they teased her more when she was in a group. She was afraid Judiath might be in the group as well.

Although Judiath lived near the school, she sometimes visited family members closer to where Grace lived. Grace ensured she looked for Judiath everywhere because Judiath was a tricky bully. Grace tried not to go outside at school except for the washroom or a drink of water. She loved playing in the schoolyard but did not do it anymore because she was afraid to be hurt by Judiath.

She tried to do her classwork without thinking of the bully or baby Jim. It was not easy. At lunch, she stayed in the classroom and worked on the chalkboard. At the end of school, she did her assignments, sharpened pencils, and waited for everyone to leave like before.

She went under the Poinsettia tree and surveyed Judiath's gate. The area seemed deserted. Grace put her pencils in her pockets and her books in her bag. She walked speedily across the field while keeping her eyes at Judiath's gate. Judiath and her friends stood near the bushes when she arrived on the roadway. They had been hidden from the schoolyard and playing field.

The gang saw Grace and came toward her. She was fearful and froze. She had nowhere to run or hide. There were about five girls with Judiath, and the whole group surrounded Grace. Judiath was face-to-face with Grace, edging nearer and nearer.

Grace was confused. Although she tried to prepare herself, she was not expecting so many people to attack her. Judiath repeatedly punched Grace in the head and face and pushed her into the bushes and down onto the asphalt. Grace fell hard, hitting her knees on the hot ground. She felt a surge of pain rush through her body. She fought to stand and catch her balance. Reaching into her pocket with her right hand, Grace took out her pencil and blindly defended herself with the sharp, yellow stick. Eyes closed, she stabbed around as she felt the other girls pulling at her uniform and striking her in the back.

Furiously, she swung the pencil up, down, left, right, and around. She screamed and shouted for them to stop. "Please, please stop, stop, please stop! You are hurting me," she pleaded.

She heard someone else scream. Grace opened her eyes and saw Judiath holding the left side of her head. One piece of a wooden pencil was sticking out of her head, and another piece was in Grace's right hand. Blood ran along Judiath's hairline and down her face. Her friends were shocked and didn't know what to do. Grace was hurt and cried when she saw the blood on Judiath's hair, forehead, and hands. This left her scared and in shock.

Grace cried as she ran home as fast as she could. Angry and in pain, she picked Jim up and held him in her arms, groaning because she was throbbing all over. She went into the kitchen and placed Jim on the floor. Grace sat on a chair and cried while she looked at her baby brother. Her knees and the palm of her left hand were scraped and had black pieces of asphalt in them. They burned like fire. The wounds on her legs throbbed with shooting pain. She was unable to stop crying.

One of the tenants called her name and asked what was wrong. She continued crying and couldn't respond. Mick had been playing outside and came in to ask her what was wrong. He tried to dry her tears, but Grace was so distraught that she brushed him away. With her face in her hands, tears on her cheek, and snot running from her nose, her shoulders shook so hard she was unable to speak.

Grace was so distressed that her little brother Jim tried to pry her hands away from her face. He looked up at her sadly as if he knew something was wrong. It was Friday afternoon; this gave Grace time to think about the trouble she was in and how to get someone to help her.

She couldn't eat because it felt like there were knots in her throat and stomach. She fed Jim and went into the room to lie down. Mick went outside to play. It must have been a while because, when Grace woke, it was dark. She heard her siblings playing in the long passageway of the house.

It was a small community, and word spread quickly among students and parents. Rose was unaware of the bullying and the damage to Judiath's head. Grace was not sure what to do or who to tell. She was afraid of the consequences.

She tried to enjoy playing, reading, laughing, and watching her mother do chores. Her ulcers were not healing and were excruciatingly painful. It was worse without proper wound care. She and her family tried to keep the sores from getting infected. Grace had no idea about infection but craved pain relief and used home remedies.

When Rose was home on weekends, they were restricted to playing in the front yard. Their mom was strict and did not socialize much with the tenants. Plus, she was busy doing things for the six of her children who lived with her. Rose was home starting on Saturday night and did a lot on Sundays. She would wash their hair, brush their teeth, bathe them, do all the laundry, and clean. Darlene helped with the cooking.

Weekends were special—Grace and her siblings were cared for with a purpose. Rose did not know how much her absence affected her children. She was not able to show up at parent-teacher meetings, get revised textbooks, stop the bullying, ensure they were clean and groomed regularly, or help them get to school on time. The children carried out these responsibilities themselves because the sitters were incapable.

They told Rose when they needed books or when parents were visiting at school, but some things did not seem important, and often the funding was unavailable. Grace shared her friends' textbooks, but it was difficult for her to learn in such a way. To learn, she had to spend time in front of the texts and visualize the content. Rose did not know much about the school system or what was required for success because she had no education.

First, she was a mother, and second, a provider. Rose was not able to assist with assignments. She didn't know how to pass on knowledge without the strap, but she did her best. Her goals were to ensure her children were comfortable and provided for. To Rose, those were the most important things. She'd been abused and did not want her children to be abused.

On Monday morning, Grace's fears returned. She headed to school but was nervous and anxious about the outcome of Friday's brawl. When she came to Judiath's gate, there were a lot of adults there. She saw her brother Dean standing with Judiath's brother, who was his friend.

She timidly walked toward the school gate. As she was about to pass the adults, Grace heard Judiath's voice say, "There she is! That is the girl who stabbed me in the head."

As someone stopped Grace, Judiath stood beside the adults with a white bandage on her head. A lady said, "Little girl, what happened last Friday? My daughter had a piece of a pencil sticking out of her head."

Grace stuttered, "Judiath and five of her friends waited for me over there." Grace pointed to the spot where the attack took place.

"They started fighting me. They slapped, punched, and pulled me into the bushes and then threw me on the road." Grace showed the lady her knees and the palm of her hand.

The lady said, "What? Speak louder, I cannot hear you," So Grace repeated what she'd said in a louder voice.

She continued, "I had my pencil in my hand, trying to stop them".

Grace had tears in her eyes as she continued, "They were hurting me, and I begged them to stop."

Judiath's mother looked authoritatively at Grace, then she looked at Judiath. She asked Judiath if this was true. Judiath nodded her head, indicating a *yes* motion. Her mother told Judiath that if she ever hurt another student, she would be in big trouble. She emphasized that Judiath was to go to school and return home immediately when school ended. Judiath was not allowed to play, walk with friends, or tease other children. She was not to stay after school but to help at home.

Judiath hung her head in shame as the other people stared at her. They asked Grace to list all the other students in the brawl. Grace listed everyone present on the day of the fight. Some of their parents talked with Judiath's mother. Grace knew all the girls were in trouble with their parents.

Dean asked Grace why she hadn't mentioned what happened while they were at home. Grace did not answer his questions. Judiath's mother indicated for Grace to continue on her way to school and she did. Judiath and her friends never bothered Grace again. It was the end of her middle school bullying. She enjoyed learning and taking care of Jim, although she was still battling pain from SCC and leg ulcers.

Judiath could not hide what had happened because of the white bandage on her head. Dean encouraged Grace to tell him if anyone tried to hurt her again. Mick stoned the girls when he saw them and warned them not to touch his sister again. Grace realized that people would listen when something went wrong. She understood that telling someone about the bullying would probably yield a better outcome.

Grace's young mind was so fearful of the pain the bullies had caused that all she wanted to do was get away and never return to the place of the event. She learned that telling someone like a family member, parent, older adult, or even a neighbour might have been more beneficial.

DOS AND DO NOTS

INFORMATION FOR PARENTS

1. Always support your child's physical, emotional, spiritual, and mental needs.
2. Ensure you understand what makes them fearful, unhappy, and scared.
3. Ensure that your child's hygienic needs are met.
4. Teach your child early on how to provide for their basic needs so they can be independent and competent.
5. Ensure that you show interest in your child's academics.
6. Attend parent-teacher meetings and check up on your child when it is least expected.
7. Ensure your child is not being bullied.
8. Teach your child not to bully others because it is wrong, hateful, and can cause irreparable brokenness.
9. If you cannot do these things for your child, ask someone you trust, and who is trustworthy, to be available to your child.
10. Do not welcome people who will assault them. Most assaults are from close family members and friends, so have a watchful eye.
11. Protect your child and listen to them because they are almost always telling the truth.
12. Trust your child over an adult because most perpetrators know that parents do not listen to their children, so they assault and abuse these young humans and get away with it.

INFORMATION FOR CHILDREN

1. Tell someone if you are being bullied or if you are not feeling well.
2. Try your best to explain what is happening.
3. Find kind people to socialize and walk with. Never walk alone if you are being bullied.
4. Ask an adult family member to accompany you because bullies are cowards and don't act when adults are around.

5. Remember that bullies are cowards who often have a difficult time at home, so do not let them take their frustration out on you. Tell someone.

6. Be honest, strong, and brave.

7. If someone is assaulting you in any way, tell someone you trust. If that person doesn't believe you, tell someone else. Do not stop talking until someone listens.

8. Be a child! Laugh, dance, sing, play, cry, learn, and talk. Most of all, have fun growing.

MY LOVES

PARENTS

Love is patient and kind; love does not envy or boast; it is not arrogant or rude. (1 Corinthians 13:4–5, ESV)

ROSE WAS FROM a large family of fifteen siblings. She was beautiful and of medium build. Grace's facial features resembled some of hers. Rose was hardworking, kind, caring, supportive, and generous—too generous. Rose loved to coordinate and had great time management and organizational skills. She was opinionated, thoughtful, shy, and worrisome. She would find things to worry about. Rose stood her ground whenever she thought something was wrong or unfair. She taught her children a lot of biblical principles and old folk tales.

She had her first baby when she was fourteen years old. Her parents were disappointed and put her out of the family home in the early stage of her pregnancy. Rose became a domestic helper who did live-in duties as a maid for a while. She moved from her home parish to live approximately a three-hour drive from her original hometown.

Rose had two children before meeting Grace's father, Lester Brown. They lived in a two-bedroom house with an outhouse. There was a shop on the front of the house. Rose and Lester did business in the shop, selling food items and liquor.

Lester's father, Ernie, felt disappointed that Lester was with Rose. He had higher expectations for his son. Ernie constantly reminded Lester that Rose wasn't good enough for him. This caused Lester to consume alcohol regularly and become an alcoholic, which led to constant conflicts with Rose. Grace was disappointed in Ernie for his disapproval of Lester because she saw the love Rose and Lester shared.

They did well in business and cared for and loved their children Nick, Andie, Dean, Darlene, Grace, and Mick. Rose and Lester lived happily at one of the crossroads where the government had installed a standpipe with running water.

The crossroad was a busy place for gossip because the standpipe was where community members gathered for water. These members fought, quarrelled, got drunk, and congregated. Rose and her family were exposed to this, which led to conflict within their home.

One night, Lester came home reeking of alcohol. Grace could hear her parents screaming insults at each other. When the argument ended, a truck drove away with everything from their home. Lester left nothing in the house. Rose was devastated. She had to give up the shop as she had no support for the six children that Lester left with her. They separated when Grace was five years old.

Grace noticed that Rose changed. She did not smile anymore and took full responsibility because she had no one else to assist. Rose moved into a big tenement yard (rooming house) because she was not financially stable. The owner of the house paid her to be the landlord. She was allowed to take most of the house and rent the rest to tenants. Rose worked hard to replace what she'd lost. Grace thought she was obsessed with proving to Lester that she could do better without him.

When Grace started having leg ulcers, Rose was worried because she was unable to control the situation. She continuously worked harder and gave money to family members to take Grace to the hospital. When no one was available, she took her.

Lester did not seem concerned. Alcoholism took over his life, and when tenants tried to explain Grace's plight, he said he would try, but nothing was ever done on his part. He did not contribute to her health in any way.

After seven years of separation, Rose conceived Jim with someone she fell in love with. Jim was an addition that significantly impacted the family. He had such sensitivity that it brought the family together in laughter and comfort.

SIBLINGS

*Strong bonds are those created and maintained
despite the differences in bloodline or background.*

Each sibling's diverse characteristics, personality, and thought processes helped to buffer Grace's harrowing life experiences. There was such variety among them all: dark, strong, handsome, beautiful, tall, slim, and medium-sized features. These qualities intertwined and created the siblings' identities. They loved each other and exhibited kindness, generosity, and honesty. They were hardworking, forgiving, skillful, playful, willing to learn, and protective of each other. Some were caring, quiet, competitive, helpful, and opinionated.

The balance of selfishness, compromise, and thoughtfulness came in packages of youthful bliss from Nick, Andie, Dean, Darlene, Mick, and Jim. These attributes clashed with each other occasionally.

Some of them were paid for being strong and hardworking. They cultivated dreams, fantasies, and successes. Grace received gifts that were treasured and hidden in her heart. She remembered special moments shared.

They were reliable, but sometimes vague and deceptive. Sometimes misguided, but they still had truthful attitudes. Promises were kept and broken. There were those whom Grace favoured, and those next in line to be favoured. The ones who would sit with her at the hospital for prolonged periods enabled her to get treatments and deal with her fear of needles.

The closeness and freedom of constant connection impacted which siblings formed and maintained their relationships. Some characteristics improved, and some continued. Some got worse and haunted them all as they grew and developed as a team bonded by bloodline.

Some kin were always busy: strapped for time, tired, unhappy, and unwilling to play or communicate much. When Grace and her siblings visited the ones who lived far away, it sometimes felt like they were imposing. This caused the visits to be less frequent and the connection strained.

The ones who loved God and were his ambassadors tried to evangelize. They invited Grace to church and taught her Bible verses. Prayers went up endlessly, seeking God on behalf of Grace's illness. They had faith that Grace's healing was around the corner. As each year advanced, however, the children of God in Grace's family formed new concepts of God's ways and plans for Grace's life. It seemed God was deaf to their endless prayers.

Rose's children tried to care for their mother. Those who were recalcitrant were severely punished for their uncouth behaviours. When Rose was away, the older siblings acted as guardians of the younger children—but they seemed stressed, troubled, and angry most of the time. They shouted in frustration for those outside to get into the house and do something more constructive than backtalking.

The older siblings took what was not theirs, showed dominance and ownership, and were territorial. Those who were employed left for work early and returned late at night. Small trinkets and items from the workplace were unfairly sold to the younger ones to rob them of their savings. The ones who had expensive taste and could not meet financial obligations borrowed without repaying. They displayed unsupportive, inconsiderate, attention-seeking, and entitled mindsets.

Some siblings found it difficult to share cherished items, which caused the others to use and take these particulars without permission. This led to conflicts and malice. Rose intervened in these situations and enforced consequences for such selfish behaviours.

The antisocial ones prevented the other siblings from making friends out of jealousy. Some were proud to form new bonds and networked in groups that practiced games like dancing, soccer, and netball.

The bad habits they picked up, such as laziness, smoking, drinking, and stealing, sometimes led to disconnection in the family and, instead, connection to those in the community with shared hobbies. Rose taught them responsibility, conflict resolution, domestic skills, and sincerity. She warned about taking a mile instead of an inch.

There were times when a sibling was jealous of Grace because of the attention she received for comfort measures. Some did not forgive her readily and held grudges against her. All their excitement, disappointments, conflicts, and agreements helped as they learned more about each other. This assisted with support and emotional regulation and helped to maintain positive mental health. Grace loved each of them in her own way.

DOS AND DO NOTS
INFORMATION FOR PARENTS

1. Know that each child has a different personality and will think differently. Do embrace their unique qualities.
2. If your child does something you do not like, try not to get angry but to discuss the issue in love.
3. Do not judge or compare siblings; instead, accommodate each one's needs.
4. Allow children to work out their conflicts in an amicable manner.

INFORMATION FOR CHILDREN

1. Show respect for your family members, especially your parents. Ask for things you need without stealing, lying, or destroying property.

2. Do not say bad things about family members because you would not like others speaking badly about you.

3. Children, respect the rules and discipline measures set by your guardians because they know best.

4. Be careful of your words when you are angry because you can't take them back, and they can hurt.

5. Do not retaliate in revenge because the consequences never turn out well.

6. Positively support your family members so they can grow and develop in a caring environment.

MOVING TO A NEW LOCATION

Stability enhances security. Ensure you build a stable environment,
a foundation to secure a future for all.

THE MORE TIME Rose spent at her restaurant, the more successful she became. This allowed her to take care of her family. She
provided what was possible but hardly ever her time. She worked
hard and had lots of friends. Grace saw her mother laughing and
becoming less stressed. She seemed freer than when Grace's
father had abandoned her and left her with nothing.

Rose had made something of herself. Her children could now
have anything they needed. This was one of her goals, and she was
flourishing. Her time and effort had paid off. When Lester left and
took everything, it had been a terrible situation. He'd moved all the
furniture out of the house they rented together. Lester had taken
this furniture to his father's place. Rose hadn't even had a stove
or bed for her children, but she didn't abandon her children. Grace
had heard her crying at night. Her attitude had been sad, and she'd
looked beaten down for a long time.

Rose had coped by getting old boards and begging work-
men to build her a restaurant in town. It was a difficult start, but
she'd gone to work early and come home late at night. Many times,
Grace and her siblings had not seen their mother. She did not know
how her mom had done it, but she had succeeded. Lots of people
loved her cooking. She was a great cook. She had mastered the
art of cooking in that old, boarded restaurant. Rose's strength was
admirable.

Rose grew happier, and she bought her kids nice things. There were numerous beds, kerosene oil stoves, clothes, shoes, and necessities for her children. There was always food and drink in the home. Rose also had a sewing machine, where she skillfully made uniforms, clothing, bedding, curtains, and other novelties.

One day, Rose's brother Jake was having trouble with his immediate family. He asked Rose to take over his successful business. Grace's uncle lived and worked in another part of the country, so Rose decided to move there with her children. This permitted Rose to be closer to her parents and siblings, as well as to work in the new business Jake had given her. Jake intended to take his children and live in the United States of America.

Rose, Andie, Dean, and Darlene packed up, and the family moved in the summertime, when school was on break. She hired a truck to take her household items to her brother's house. They were all excited for this journey. She had taken the kids on such journeys many times before but only to visit her mom. Rose had no family members in the town where she and the children lived. With no support system, she'd suffered a lot of abuse and exploitation.

Rose's mother lived about ten kilometres from her brother Jake. This relocation would benefit her and the kids because her family would be close. She had fifteen siblings: eight brothers and seven sisters. Most of them were in foreign countries like England, the United States of America, and Canada.

When they arrived at Jake's home, they saw that it was on a slope. It was beautiful and clean, with electricity and available water. The dirt in the yard was black. They saw flowers all around for edging and a white picket gate. The house had two bedrooms and a living room, kitchen, unfinished washroom, verandah, medium-sized shop to the right side of the entrance, and big dance hall, which was attached to the house with a passageway that ran in between.

The house was painted in white, with red floors. There were three big bay windows with louvers on both ends, in the living room and master bedroom. The other areas also had louver windows. The house had three main entrances. Anyone could walk through the shop to get into the house. There was an outhouse. The dance hall was not painted, but the shop was brown-coloured.

Inside the house, they found a fridge, deep freezer, record player, television, sofa, gas stove, and video cassette recorder (VCR). These were things they'd never had at the old house. Back then, they'd had kerosene oil stoves, lamps, and radios. They'd played outside, bathed in a wash tub, and caught water from the concrete tank or the pipe. The family had never stored food but cooked regularly. Previously, they'd spent less time indoors, so a sofa had not been necessary. As before, though, they continued to bathe in a washtub outside and use the outhouse toilet.

All around them were fruit trees: mango, naseberry, banana, coconut, lime, plum, sugar cane, orange, and apple. There were no tenants and no red dirt, and at the side of the house, there was a big black water tank they had to pay the government to fill. The structure was firm, the walls intact, and the land prosperous.

The nearest neighbour was about three hundred metres away. About five or six graves rested in front of the gate on the other side of the road. A fence surrounded the land. It was less chaotic, quieter, and smaller. It provided more closeness with the family. Rose was always home, since the business operated at the front of the house.

Darlene was not able to move with the rest of the family. She was in the ninth grade and had two more years to graduate, after which she would join the others. She stayed with her brother Nick and his wife and children for that time. Darlene was missed for those years because they had never been apart before that move.

Grace was twelve years old at the time of their relocation. She was excited to live in another part of the island—in a different town, near her favourite Aunt Nina and her cousins. This aunt and the cousins had usually visited in the summer, but their trips were never long. When they'd visited Grace's home, the whole family had enjoyed laughing, reminiscing, and feasting together. Grace had prayed they would visit every summer, but her aunt and cousins rarely came.

Moving to another parish was beneficial for Grace. The warmer weather enhanced her comfort level. In addition, the SCD professional and research team clinic at one of the biggest hospitals in Montego Bay was about fifteen kilometres away. It was a specialized sickle cell (SC) clinic with knowledgeable doctors and nurses.

This clinic offered monthly SCD monitoring, research, quarterly blood test monitoring, better wound care, wound care products, and wound care monitoring. The specialists prescribed antibiotics when her ulcers were infected, and the clinic covered all medications. The nurses educated Grace about sickle cell disease in such a way that she could understand what was happening and how the sickling was inherited and genetically tested. They taught her the benefits of diet, rest, medication, and research. She learned about wounds, necrotic areas on the skin, infections, and monthly checkups.

Grace had not had proper health care management where she'd lived before. She was happy because now someone cared enough to think about her illness as well as how to help other people living with SCD. At this clinic, Grace learned she was never to take a blood transfusion, despite her hemoglobin levels. Rose always ensured that Grace visited the SCD clinic every month.

By the time Grace celebrated her thirteenth birthday—just before the school year in July—she was limping terribly from sores on both ankles. The constriction in her right foot had caused her left foot to be longer than the right. Her right heel could hardly touch the ground because it was agonizing to walk normally.

There was no normalcy in Grace's painful little life. The changes to the body structure in her legs were obvious. She dreaded what others would do and say in this new environment. The fear, anxiety, and grief she felt starting a new school were underestimated.

It was difficult for Grace to find comfortable footwear that accommodated both feet. Her mother bought beautiful, well-designed shoes for her, but her feet wouldn't fit because of their tenderness and deformity. They were either too tight or too flat; either they had high edges or didn't support her bandages; some were too close, and others not close enough. It was an exhausting search, and nothing worked. Grace promised to wear the best and nicest shoes when her feet were healed.

Her new school had a shift system that switched every year. One year she was on the morning shift, the next she would be on the evening. Or one term the shift would change. Grace was well advanced in her classes and had excellent grades. She'd learned a lot from her old school, which was advanced compared to the new one.

Grace came first in her grades and did not know that being a brilliant student would become a risk factor for being bullied. She tried to attend school every day, but it was impossible with her wounds and pain. After going to school for two or three days, her feet would be so swollen and painful that Grace had to stay in bed for the remainder of the week to recuperate. The walking journey to school was thirty to forty-five minutes back and forth. Sometimes she took the bus home when it got late or when her ulcers were brutally hurting.

At times, the bus was so packed that there was no available standing space. She would stand on one foot, and when it got tired and achy, she'd switch legs. The bus took forever to reach her destination. The long time spent standing, and the people stepping on each other and shoving, pushing, or squeezing one another, caused excruciating pain to creep up her legs and into her body. Her entire body felt crushed in agony, and misery filled her heart. The pain crept into every cell and ignited them like a flame torch.

The choices were to walk or take the bus. Either option caused unyielding pain that wracked her body to pieces. It was like an explosion building in the cells of her organs, bones, and joints and causing a volcanic rapture from toes to head. The pain took an eternity to subside, even after taking Panadol, Phenic, Cafenol, or Aspirin. These were the only pills available. No one knew the levels of her suffering. No one seemed to understand her plight or her journey through this torturous life. She tried to find hope in the other students who seemed to be enjoying themselves.

Grace observed their activities and dreamed of being able to play again. She sat in corners, wondering what it would be like to run, jump, skip, swim, dance, and walk without being plagued. Sometimes she could visualize a world without pain or distress, and she prayed silently in her heart. Sometimes she had visions of herself walking in nicely designed shoes without limping or tiptoeing—without aches—but with confidence, pride, joy, and comfort. She could hear her heart whisper, "You have arrived! You have conquered."

When Grace was sick, she was sad and bored during the recuperating phase. Reading helped her state of mind. She delved into books—the bigger the book, the more the comfort. Her mother was home all the time and knew her pain. Rose understood the woes Grace was going through because she heard her cries. The sobs were constant. Grace saw the concerned looks on Rose's face and tried to pretend she was fine, but Grace's eyes told a different story.

The move to another parish had reduced Rose's entrepreneurial success. Jake's shop wasn't as busy as her previous restaurant. The community members thought the new strangers shouldn't be supported, especially since Jake's in-laws had been expecting to get the shop. Rose taking over the shop caused conflict and separation between Jake's family and his in-laws. There were continuous battles, curses, and threats toward Grace's family.

Rose became unhappy. To keep up a motherly perspective, she sang, prayed, attended churches, went to the market, read her

Bible, washed and pressed the clothes, cooked, and watched television. This was good for Grace and her siblings because now they had the motherly support that had not been as readily available at their old place. Rose was able to monitor her children more closely. Her children attended school with clean, well-pressed uniforms, were fed healthy meals, and were organized.

Everything had changed, Mick and Dean were in soccer groups. Grace watched television and read. Dean played music, and Mick played video games. Andie went to work and had a girlfriend. The closeness and creativity they'd used to make games and play together were gone. They started living separate lives because of their different activities and school shifts but always reunited at the end of the day.

Only Jim and Rose were home when Grace was sick. She was allowed to do anything that made her happy and pain free, which was never possible. When she had company, she cried inside. It was brutal to contain the affliction internally. Grace went to her bed and cried alone when the discomfort was uncontrollable.

DOS AND DO NOTS

INFORMATION FOR CHILDREN

1. Ensure you know your surroundings and how to find safety in an emergency.
2. Remember, not everyone will like you, and that is okay.
3. Practice treating everyone with kindness even when they do not treat you with kindness.
4. New locations might be different from old places; make the best of the situation.
5. Do not lose hope no matter what you are going through. There are great things ahead.
6. Explore strategies that bring comfort and use them when in need.
7. Find positive distractive methods to soothe your mind.

8. If you are not okay, say you are not. Do not lie to people about your well-being.

9. There are different social groups available that can be a support system.

10. Ask for advice from people who are experienced. Do not suffer alone.

11. No matter what, love and respect who you are and strive for better.

DIFFERENT LOCATION,
NEW BULLIES

The Holy Spirit helps humans to intertwine and relocate so they can support each other and evolve.

AT THE NEW school, the bullying was worse. Grace was bullied for many reasons. Her sores constantly drained and wet the dressings within minutes after wound care. Although she wore blue socks and black plastic shoes with her uniforms, the drainage was obvious on her socks. Yet Grace was beautiful, despite her limitations, which was an additional reason to be bullied.

Some students believed that a stranger from another parish and country school should not come first or do better than the regular students. These students did not know how hard Grace worked academically, especially when she couldn't attend school. She did double the work and studied harder in preparation for sick days. She would work far ahead of the students in her class, and it made her an excellent pupil. Grace also studied to divert her thoughts from the pain, hurt, and grief that was always there.

Certain students, such as Dora, Tina, Marcia, Chrisy, and Oneil, bullied Grace constantly. They lived in the same community and would wait for Grace after school. The bullying was less vicious when she took the bus. These individuals did not want the adults on the bus to know the troublemakers they were. When they walked home, they teased, said cruel things about her, called her names, and threw stones, papers, and twigs at her. They slapped and pushed her, and sometimes Grace fell because of her balance issue.

Their behaviours scared Grace. Her heart would palpitate loudly in her chest; she cried silently and secretly wiped tears away. These harassments happened every time she went to school. All of the bullies were in the same grade, but only a few were in Grace's classroom.

Dora was the worst of all. She seemed so unhappy most times, and Grace never saw her smile. Dora teased Grace and said bad things about her, planning to fight her many times after school. Grace was unable to physically defend herself, especially from Dora. Grace defended herself by using hurtful and feisty words. These cruel words caused Dora to be outraged.

Grace was dreadfully afraid of Dora. When she slapped Grace in the face, it left her fingerprints all over. Dora planned to harm Grace, so Grace didn't want to attend school. When she did, she hid in the classrooms, refusing to go to the washroom or take breaks. Grace was nervous and shied away from these bullies. She stayed on the school grounds until the evening bus left, thinking the children would likely ride home on it.

Grace thought Dora had taken the bus. She slowly walked to the bus stop and scrutinized the environment to ensure Dora was not there. It was late afternoon, about 5:00 p.m. School had ended at 3:00 p.m., so Grace was surprised to see Dora hiding under the bus stop and waiting for her.

Grace tried to run back into the schoolyard, but Dora was faster. Dora grabbed her and used her fists to pound on her. She slapped her face and tore her uniform. Grace fell to her knees on the gravel road, covered her face, and screamed in pain. Mercilessly, Dora rained slaps, fists, and kicks on Grace.

All the other students and teachers from the morning shift had left. The ones on the evening shift were in class. No one was there to assist Grace. She felt the heat on her skin, stinging and swelling her face, neck, and head. When she heard another bus coming, she got up off her knees, ran toward the stop zone, and got on the bus, crying all the way home. She was in so much pain from the physical assault and leg ulcers, she felt she'd go insane.

Grace sat at the end of her street and cried when she disembarked the bus. She tried to refocus and recompose herself. She lived opposite the street that Dora had to take home. Her brother Dean came down the street and inquired what was wrong, so she told him that Dora attacked her at school. When she showed him her face, neck, and head—these areas had wheals—and the red, swollen areas showing Dora's hands and fingerprints, Dean was furious. He knew it took a lot for Grace to cry, and he could see that Grace was sad, torn, and beaten.

He told Grace that later they were going down to where Dora lived to slap her back. Grace started to cry more because she was terrified of Dora. She told her brother she didn't want to do it. Dean was firm about his decision to fight back. He looked at her with sternness in his eyes and disappointment on his face. Grace knew he was serious.

Later that evening, Dean took Grace down Spring Road to face the girl who had beaten his sister. When they arrived at the Spring Road entrance, Dora was standing there with a bucket filled with water. Dean took Grace over to her and directed his questions to Dora.

"Why did you beat up my sister? What did she do to you? Why did you slap her all over? Why were you bullying her?" Dean shouted in anger.

Dora looked at Dean without saying anything. Dean took his sister's hand, walked closer to the girl, and demanded that Grace slap Dora the same way Dora had done to Grace earlier. Grace's heart was beating out of her chest. She was nervous and tried hard to catch her breath. She knew that Dora would hurt her at school again. Grace could not explain this to Dean, who insisted that Grace slap back this evil-looking tyrant.

Grace was reluctant but could not tell Dean about the dread and fear that lingered in her heart. She sensed that Dora saw this and was secretly basking in her power to dominate the life of her victim. Dean held Grace's right hand and pulled her nearer to the young bully. He physically lifted Grace's right hand and swung it forcefully across Dora's left cheek since Grace resisted doing it willingly. He told Dora that every time she beat up his sister, he would return the favour right where she stood.

Dean got angry and swore at Dora, who just stood and stared, quiet, tall, and angry. Dora doubled the size of Grace in height and body mass. There was a look of vengeance in Dora's eyes as she looked at Grace and her brother. It was difficult for Grace to imagine the torture that Dora would be inflicting on her at school.

This strong, heavy-handed girl, who did not seem affected by the slap she received from Grace would not let this humiliation go. From the look of her attitude, she would avenge that slap at all costs. Dean told her that if she bullied his sister again, he would go directly to her parents to complain.

Dora continued to fight and terrorize Grace at school. They fought and exchanged hateful words until school became unbearable for Grace. Then Dora stopped the abuse unexpectedly. Grace wondered if maybe Dean had spoken to her family about the bullying. Most families are afraid of the shame and guilt associated with the harm their family members cause other people. Families try to live respectably and charitably in their communities.

Suddenly, Dora stopped attending school. She was not seen in the community again, so the bullying from her finally ended. Grace did not know or care what had happened but rejoiced from the relief.

After a while, though, Tina, Marcia, Chrisy, and Oneil took over where Dora had left off. The three girls watched while Oneil teased and called Grace names like "sore-foot gal." Grace used words to defend herself, which got Oneil angry. They were walking up a slope when Oneil ran toward her, jumped into the air, and landed kicks into Grace's chest. She fell hard, backward onto the road. Her elbows and other body parts were scratched, scraped, and bruised. She cried for the rest of the two-kilometre walk home. Her chest ached where the kicks had landed, as did her arms, legs, and buttocks.

Grace was sad because she was physically, emotionally, and mentally sick. Her spirit was broken by the children who were unkind and evil. She reported the incident to Rose, who went straight to the grandparents and parents of Oneil. They apologized for his behaviour, and from that day on, Oneil never teased or assaulted Grace again.

DOS AND DO NOTS

INFORMATION FOR PARENTS

1. Pay attention when your child's attitudes and behaviours change.
2. Protect your child from being bullied.
3. Talk to your child about mistreatment from others: what it looks like, what it might sound like, and how to have an open conversation.
4. Trust your child's words and speak to the parents of the bullies.
5. Do not repeat what your child confided in you to the person about whom they reported.
6. Observe your child and how others interact with them. Talk about fairness, justice, and equality.

INFORMATION FOR CHILDREN

1. Tell your guardians about any mistreatment you might be experiencing.
2. You might feel intimidated and scared to report the bully but report the mistreatment to an adult.

3. Do not forget that you are beautiful and handsome, and your self-confidence is important.
4. Tell yourself frequently how worthy and deserving you are and that no one can take that from you.
5. Do not underestimate your potential. Ask for help and always do your best.

PLAYING AND SCHOOLING

When there is internal damnation, education will be a minute achievement compared to pain and loss.

GRACE WAS HAVING difficulties at her new school in part because of her difference in parish dialect. Her pronunciations of some words, like *yellow,* sounded weird to the other students and teachers.

She had newly revised textbooks, however, and did her assignments effectively. At the school there was a library. There were different teachers, such as the school nurse, an agriculturalist, a mechanic, and a counsellor. She went to grade 7, where there were many sections, such as 7-1, 7-2, 7-3, all the way to 7-7. Those who did excellent schoolwork and were in the top thirty from grade 6 went to grades 7-1 and 7-2. These classes were the top in their grades. Grace was in 7-1.

It was different from her previous school. She avoided classes such as physical education, economics, and food and beverage because she was constantly teased. She was not physically fit and had pain after exertion.

Grace went from the classroom to the tuck shop and then back to class. Grade 9 was easier than the other grades she'd done. The students were more settled and serious with their studies.

Little to no bullying, odious name-calling, or envy existed in the ninth grade. Being bullied was something Grace had gotten used to and was able to manage. The anger built into Grace's system from past cruelties surpassed all the bullies. If a student reported an assault to a homeroom teacher, they could be kicked out of school. The teacher would send for their parents, and it was not a good sign for parents to be seen at the principal's office.

In the ninth grade, the teachers prepared the students for the tenth and eleventh grades heading toward graduation. If they did not do well, it would be unfortunate for them and their family members who had worked hard to send their children to school. Everyone tried to make their parents proud by receiving a graduation certificate.

Grace was able to breathe a little easier. She had friends in the ninth grade and students who wanted to be with her in class. It was still difficult to deal with the ulcer pain. When she played too much, there was pain all over her body that radiated from her wound to other parts of her body. There were also aches in her bones and joints. The pain was uncomfortable and debilitating at times.

Most times, Grace sat in class and did classwork. Physical Education was mandatory, but Grace had a grueling time with exercise. The teachers were undereducated about her illness, unable to protect her from sickle cell crisis (SCC), and not taking Grace seriously when she tried to explain her condition to them. In addition, they would not listen because they were adults. The cultural norms and mannerisms of the school expected students to obey all rules.

Grace desired to play with friends, succeed in school, walk without pain, have normal legs, and be a healthy child. Her hopes and dreams were so gigantic, it felt like they were bursting through her whole being. Her fantasies soared beyond the skies, past the stars, and stretched to eternity.

Her illness had given her yearnings that took wings beyond the school walls and into the open world—yearnings to function, live, love, earn, provide, gain, and help. She saw and felt something "out there" that her wounds prevented her from achieving. Grace needed healing before everything inside her exploded into unrealized potential. She knew such aspirations started within the school system, so learning to bring out her full potential was important.

Although she had hopes and dreams, her surroundings left her in woe, isolation, and a lack of authenticity, especially at school. Those who were meant to protect, school, and encourage her kept shouting at her and making insulting comments like, "Learn to pronounce your Ys properly! If you cannot, you will never read in class again."

The descriptions and furious words that some of her teachers used caused Grace embarrassment that eventually brought shyness, shame, and guilt to her self-esteem. The social and art classes were the worst. She was prohibited from reading in English class, so Grace focused on the classes where her teachers provided positive reinforcement and goal outcomes.

Grace's favourite classes were Science, Clothing and Textiles, Mathematics, and Music. She liked Agriculture but was unable to stand for long periods. She strived and excelled in the sciences. Her science, maths, and music teachers were lovely and kind. They saw the potential and encouraged Grace to succeed.

Grace's clothing and textiles teacher most times shouted at her to lift her feet and stop dragging her shoes across the floor. If only she knew the effort it took Grace to lift her sore feet up and off the floor. If only she understood the pain that jolted through her body with such a simple act of movement. If only she could experience the stinging, heaviness, electric shocks, struggles, and fiery sensations each step caused. Grace's feet on the ground ached just as much as when they were off the ground.

"Lift your feet off the ground, Grace, and stop dragging your shoes on the floor," was just one of the annoyances of people who advised her without knowledge.

There was not much playtime at school. Grace's small stature, sluggishness, and timidity caused her to be excluded from the drama team, dance, and other classes that required physical participation. She could not do some of the physical stunts needed to win competitions.

Grace loved track and field but was unable to participate in a race. The cheerleading team was where she fit in best and where she enjoyed herself because she sat, sang, clapped, shouted, and cheered the team on. These activities still ignited each cell and every nerve ending with intense, shooting pain that screamed for release, but she needed to be involved in something.

The best playtime was at home with her siblings. At home, their outside games included hopscotch, Chinese skipping, going to the rivers or springs, picking various fruits with long sticks, and comparing different types of fruits and their tastes. This was fun because she loved fruits like star apples, rose apples, naseberries, mangoes, pears, apples, guineups, jackfruits, plums, and guavas, but she also loved the time spent with her loved ones throughout the year.

Indoors, it was board games, books, hide-and-seek, cooking, chatting with neighbours, videos, and cards. It was fun to play competitive games with her siblings. All of them would win occasionally. Grace preferred indoor games because she did not have the stamina, strength, or drive to run around competitively. Her pain was less intense when she was off her feet.

People say playing and schooling are integral to a child's life, but this is not the case when the child's overall distress is stealing their joy. Grace learned that after playing excessively, aggressively, and for long periods of time, her bones and joints hurt uncontrollably. Traditional and medical comfort measures were inadequate and nonfunctional for the significance of her trauma.

Grace promised to take care of herself and avoided activities that aggravated a crisis in the cells. She realized the healing, inflicting, rehealing, and rehurting processes were constant and that there must be a break in the process to stop this vicious cycle. Grace tried to learn how to train her mind to deal with her SCD and SCC.

Socializing with friends who came to her house was enjoyable. It took Grace's mind off her troubles for short periods. They talked and had restful playtimes without the painful physical hassle and bustle. She was learning to play safely and healthily, and to avoid the exhaustion, torment, and suffering that infuriated her bones and joints.

Grace's friends, siblings, and mother reminded her consistently that she did not have to play like other children but had to take it easy. They encouraged her to do simpler activities like reading and sewing. She used her mother's sewing machine to create extraordinary pieces. It took a lot of willpower to complete a design. Sewing caused her a significant amount of pain because of the vibration of the electrical motor her foot operated.

She watched cartoons and movies on television, did assignments, sat on the verandah, and watched people as they went by, ensuring she enjoyed her childhood with happiness and comfort. These activities reduced ineffective pain management and encouraged conducive playtime to enhance healing, health, and wellness. A comfortable and pain-free lifestyle enabled her to enjoy her friends and family better. She experienced peace and serenity, with less stress, when she stayed in one place.

DOS AND DO NOTS
INFORMATION FOR PARENTS

1. Help your child with SCD to find interesting and safe pain-free activities.
2. Get involved in these activities to keep the game interesting and fun because children love it when their parents are involved in their developmental goals.
3. Find new ways to introduce different programs into your child's life that encourage bone and joint health, such as daily exercises of at least 15-30 minutes.
4. Monitor your child during exercises or ask someone to monitor them. When the child looks tired, encourage them to stop.

Overindulgence can cause joint and bone pain which can be hard to control.

5. Know that pain from SCD can lead to other complications such as hemolysis of blood cells causing collection of dead blood cells in the liver and gallbladder leading to stomach aches and other aches and pains (Smith, 2024).

6. Know when your child looks healthy or is not doing well so early treatment can be provided.

INFORMATION FOR CHILDREN

1. Tell your parent(s) when you are not doing well so speedy care can be provided.

2. Do exercises that help you heal and not the ones that cause your body to ache from consistent pain. Just build your strength and do not overdo the tasks.

3. Stop the activities when you feel tired. You do not have to go to school if you are not doing well. Ask your friends or teachers to have your assignments delivered so you can keep up with classes.

4. There is a possibility that you will be bullied due to prejudice against physical changes. Tell someone when you are being bullied. Know that the person(s) who bullies you has problems that have nothing to do with you.

5. Remember that you are brave and strong in dealing with SCD and SCC, so be confident, resilient, and have high self-esteem because you are great.

6. If you cannot play contact sports, use another medium like a computer to set up contact sports games where you can play online.

7. When playing online, be careful to avoid predators that could harm you.

8. Wherever you go, be aware and careful so that you can stay safe.

9. Remember, you are much healthier and happier when you have self-control over your mind.

COPING WITH PAIN AND STAGNANCY

When stability enhances security, it leads to internal and external relaxation and harmony.

IT WAS SORROWFUL for Grace to stay home, resting in a stable position with her feet elevated. It drove her insane when her siblings and mother insisted that she rest. Grace was vibrant, at least in her mind, and needed friends nearby to stabilize her thoughts. The more she stayed alone, the more isolation gripped at her soul. She questioned herself, wondering why she should suffer like this. Why sickle cell? Boredom got the better of her when she was alone, and questions flooded her mind. When will it be over? Will it be normal again? And what would it be like without overbearing wounds?

In the community, Grace had bubbling and cheerful friends who came to visit, friends like Cathrine, Patrice, Faye, and Clifford. Sometimes when she laughed and talked about community gossip, she forgot her dilemma. At times, Grace's friends got busy with chores, school, and employment. Movies became her favourite pastime, especially comedies and cartoons.

Grace watched other children do various activities that enticed her. They ran around with their arms open, reminding her of free birds in total happiness. The looks on their faces jolted a need in Grace's stomach. She longed to play activities that enhanced her muscle strength so she could tolerate the pain. Each time she tried, though, pain shot from her feet and spread throughout her body. This caused a sense of dreariness due to her limitations. She was happy for her siblings and friends who were able to play their games.

Grace cheered them on. She never felt she could wish her pain on any of them—the pain she experienced by the second, minute, hour, and day. She couldn't imagine anyone she knew having to endure the disease she carried. She always wanted the best for them. Yet for herself, she hungered to have freedom of movement, or to return to her early childhood, or to jump ahead to a pain-free future.

Grace was academically brilliant and would help others with their assignments. She was not satisfied to simply live with her coping skills. They were too restrictive. She was tired of the constant reminders to elevate her legs. Was there no other way of staying healthy? She was sick of being told to do something different from what she wanted to do. She thought she would never heal because she didn't know how to stay steady. Grace wanted to play and do what others liked her to do—she wanted both her worlds to meet.

Grace believed there was so much more to achieve in the world and more to life than an illness. She knew that her sickle cells and various complications hindered her from shining. Her disease took away her energy and joy and sucked at her life like a leech. She continued to pray for better days. How soon that would be, she had no idea.

DOS AND DO NOTS
INFORMATION FOR PARENTS

1. Focus on your child and know when they are not experiencing adequate mental health. Depression can go unrecognized in children because they hide it well.

2. Do not push them for answers if they cannot answer the question themselves. Just support them and get community assistance in monitoring them safely.

3. Understand that young minds do not know how to deal with severe changes maturely. Embrace them with compassion and care.

4. Teach your child how to cope with pain and trauma positively. Exhaust every possibility available.

5. Speak life into your child and constantly pray for them. Let them know the world is at their fingertips and is achievable.

INFORMATION FOR CHILDREN

1. Remember your parents are there to assist with problems you are experiencing. Trust them, confide in them, and take their advice.

2. When there is fear, anxiety, and uncertainty, speak to your parents because they are wise and will try to assist.

3. Speak kindly and do not be disrespectful, especially to those who care for and love you. Value the trust they've placed in you because it is hard to rebuild.

WOUND CARE

Which man is worth saving? The physical? The mental? The emo-
tional? The spiritual? Or the financial? Each person must decide
for themselves which is most important.

THERE WAS ONE thing Grace feared more than bullying, and that
was wound care. The wound on her right leg was about 4.5 inches
by 2.5 inches. The one on the left leg was 3.5 inches by 3 inches.
This included the periwound. The edges were rolled and severely
tender. It took hours for the dressing change to be completed.

Grace was terrified every time the daily dressing change
needed to be done. She was agitated and anxious, knowing that
with every second she peeled off the old dressing, there would be
severe agony. Delaying the wound care extended the trauma. Daily,
Grace boiled water with a little salt and let it cool. She went around
the side of the house with gauze, clean bandages, cotton balls, and
the cooled saltwater.

Grace made herself comfortable on a large rock with a tow-
el on it. She knew it would take hours before the task was done.
Her heart was beating a familiar tune like a slow death that was
approaching. She knew that her heart would be in torture for hours
once she started the dressing change. The palpitations pounded in
her teeth, mouth, belly, ears, and head. Pounded like a huge stone
on the hot earth… boom, boom, boom, boom.

The pain seemed to escape through screams that lingered
within secret places of her soul. The bandages stuck to the gauze,
and the gauze to the wounds. She soaked, then slowly peeled
away the wet gauze, screaming in pain and swearing under her
breath. She felt no anger but simply a yearning for help.

The old and new dressings caused the same amount of excruciating misery. Grace wet the dressings frequently, hoping they would be easier to remove. She got the same result—despair. Each time she removed an area of the gauze, she waited for other sections to loosen.

It seemed to take forever. The tears in Grace's eyes reflected on her face, and her heart trembled. When the old dressings came off, the meshed gauze left indentations of little holes on the surface of the wounds. She slowly cleaned the wounds with the cotton balls and makeshift saline water. Every stroke caused her to clench her teeth as if to grind away the grief. Everything she did to and for the wound caused blinding grief. Every cell in her body vibrated with needle sticks and shivers. She felt the sensation in each cell individually, as they burst out in tumult.

After every dressing change, Grace lay down with both feet in her hands, caressing and willing the anguish away. As the years went by, the dressing changes only got worse. She wondered how long she had to endure. How long could her heart take the disappointment? How long would it take for her situation to be resolved?

After the wound care, it took hours for the torment to subside. Nothing she did worked. Deep inside, it felt as if strings in her heart were silently tearing away—she was overwhelmed by stress and felt completely out of control. Discontentment and hopelessness drowned out her dreams and desires. Yet she still had faith and high hopes of getting well.

Grace tried numerous therapies to keep her childish self alive. People in and around the community recommended several things for wound healing. She was encouraged by the SCD clinic to use papaya, a natural wound care treatment. She got fresh papaya from the tree in their backyard, grated it, and prepared it as a papaya paste. Grace organized herself to get the wound care done. She was excited to see how this product worked in wound healing. She followed the wound care routine, cleaned the wound, and then applied the papaya paste.

Grace's soul ripped apart as the sap in the fruit stung and burned her for the entire day. She cried, groaned, and swore not to try any other recommended treatment. The pain was unbearable. She was bedridden for the whole day. She slept periodically throughout the pain while trying to distract herself with television and illusive dreams.

The next day, the surfaces of her wound beds had tiny, sloughed areas everywhere. The edges were swollen and more tender than usual. Grace decided not to use this treatment again.

Eventually, her promise not to try another recommended treatment was forgotten out of desperation. She was willing to try the antibiotic dust from capsules. People swore that they worked to heal wounds. Grace bought some red-and-black capsules from the compound pharmacy in the city. She was excited to try this.

The wound care process was carried out, and she opened the capsules carefully to expose the white powder, then dusted it on the sores. There was no burning. It felt smooth, soothing, and comfortable. She was enjoying the feeling and did not have to go to bed as an invalid from wound care agony. She relished that day and anticipated what her wounds would look like at the next dressing change.

The next day, after the wound care was finally done, she found dried crusted surfaces that could not be cleaned properly because of the crusts. There were spaces between the dried areas with pockets between the crust and wound bed. When parts of the crusts were peeled away, there was a glass-like film over the wounds and a pinkish colour underneath.

It was challenging for Grace to remove the film and see what the actual wounds looked like. She didn't know what to use on the ulcer, so she opted to sprinkle more capsule dust because it hadn't hurt her like the other treatments. She only sprinkled the small areas directly on the sore beds because the crusted areas were already hard with old white powder.

The next day, after the second treatment of capsule powder, the crusted areas of the sores were dried and thickened. The pockets between the crusts and wounds was larger with small, chipped pieces stuck to the old dressings. The edges of the wound showed no signs of healing like they had before. The big difference was that the gauze directly on the wound was easier and less painful to remove.

The wounds felt stiff from the dryness. Although this dressing did not hurt as much, Grace knew she needed a different product to help maintain wound integrity: something with moisture balance, not too wet or too dry. She tried to detach all the crusts from the surfaces, but it took days. The most soothing treatment turned out to be ineffective. This was a dream destroyer.

The Sickle Cell Clinic provided Grace with wound care items each month. She made a saline solution and did the wet-to-dry routine. This was where she put moist, saline-soaked gauze over the sores and wrapped them in place after the wounds were cleansed. The torturous and time-consuming process restarted, as did the nightmares.

This went on for a while until someone told Grace she shouldn't have used the black-and- red capsules. Instead, it should have been the orange-and-red capsules. The individual swore this colour helped their wounds get better. Grace was encouraged to try this. Although she'd had terrible experiences with previous therapies, she was willing to have one more hope. She went to the chemist and got her new capsules.

She followed the process of her wound care, and at the end of cleaning, she opened the capsules and put the powder on her sores. At that moment, her life changed. This yellow powder on her sores burned without mercy. She had never felt anything burn like that; she screamed and fell off the rock onto the ground. She got up and ran for some cool boiled water to wash this burning agent out of her sores. That was the worst mistake of all. The wet powder stuck in her wounds and stung even worse.

She went out to the veranda and rolled on the floor in agony. Her sister, who had joined them three years prior, came to look at what was happening and saw that Grace had used a burning agent in her wound again. Darlene advised her to take some pain medication. Grace had already done that, and nothing was working.

Grace cried so hard that some of the neighbours came to see what was happening. They had compassion in their eyes, but no one could help the situation. The pain lasted for a long time that day, longer than usual. She took many painkillers, whimpered from exhaustion, and crawled on her hands and knees through the living room and kitchen toward her bedroom.

On her bed, Grace rolled from side to side, rubbed her legs up and down, and held her feet in her hands. She prayed for mercy and willed herself to sleep. When she was awake, every second felt like guitar strings ripping apart in her heart. She felt death creeping upon her. Grace gasped for breath, trying to settle her heart and the ripping sensation she felt in her chest.

She realized then that pain could kill her. For hours, the powder in her sores cleaved to every cell on the wound beds like leeches. It felt like demons were clawing through the wounds to her soul. There was nothing to stop the burn. Grace fought to be brave and face the torture, but it was too much.

Grace stayed in bed for the entire day and used a pail at her bedside to urinate. Luckily, she didn't need a bowel movement, or she would have had to use the pail for that as well. She felt reduced to her lowest point. Disabled. No matter what position her feet were in, they hurt so badly that she was losing her mind.

She knew that no one should be in such pain. No one should have a God who claimed he cared and yet find themselves in that much pain. She realized that her faith was fading, her dreams were dying, and her hopes were turning to darkness. She realized there was no way out of the turmoil.

She looked through the window and saw the brightly lit ball of sunshine pouring into the room. In the rays she felt a sense of anger, hatred, resentment, and fear. The peace she'd had was broken into a million pieces, like dust particles. The joy of a brighter tomorrow collapsed as she buried her face in the pillow and wept. She wept for a lost little girl, a damaged teenager, and a destitute future.

She cried for everything she'd lost that day. The month that marked her fifth year of suffering with open sores approached, and she remembered what the doctors had said: She would not live past eighteen. In that moment, Grace decided God was no longer a part of her life. She swore that vicious day that God did not care and neither did she.

Grace knew that the agony she'd felt the day before could not be good for her wounds. She just stayed in bed with the gloom in her heart, the gloom that had replaced everything. She wept softly and silently. She felt robbed of a childhood, and now she was almost seventeen years old. She felt robbed of her teenage years. She realized she had nothing and could have nothing. Her desire for healing ended.

Two days after the red-and-orange capsule incident, Grace decided to do her wound care. She did not care what they looked like anymore, but the wounds must be cleaned. They were dark-red to black in colour. The surfaces looked burned, scorched, or worse. She came to terms with the fact that she had sores and a responsibility to treat them because they were a part of the whole.

Grace followed her wound care routine. When she felt like they were infected, she saw the practitioners at the Sickle Cell Clinic. Sometimes they gave her antibiotics or told her they were not infected. From then on, she never talked about her sores to anyone except her doctors. This matter was a private and sensitive one.

The incident with the red-and-orange capsules put a stop to all conversations between her and other people, as well as between her and God. Everything she'd used had hurt her, even soaking her feet in seawater. Occasionally she felt sparks of hope, but she quickly and quietly quashed them to avoid having too much hope.

DOS AND DO NOTS

INFORMATION FOR PARENTS

1. Help your child with adjunctive medicine such as homeopathic therapies.
2. Listen to your child's distress and be silent during the process.
3. Always pray for your child because they occasionally lose hope and faith.
4. Try to let the child do what they want even though they might not feel well. Sometimes they feel like they are missing out which worsens the situation.

INFORMATION FOR CHILDREN

1. You may not have an open wound but are experiencing something that distresses you. Research it and see how you can get assistance with it.
2. If you have an open wound, do not feel ashamed. Explore different wound care options and don't forget to keep your hope alive.
3. It can be devastating to experience unrelieved pain. Use all the resources you find for adequate pain control.
4. Take note of what works for you and tell your healthcare providers so they can accommodate your needs.
5. Remember that people are trying to help, so have an open mind and assist them.

GRADUATION

Some people underestimate the impact of education, but appropriate knowledge enhances wisdom for decision-making.

ALTHOUGH SHE FELT she had no future, Grace still thought about her high school graduation and what she wanted to do. Every day, she went to school and picked up Jim as usual. Every school day, Grace went past the furniture shop on the main street in town. Normally, she saw a boy who worked there come to the storefront to watch her as she passed. He always stared at her and indicated that he wanted to talk. But Grace was shy, and she had not had a boyfriend before. Still, the boy religiously waited for her when she used the main street route. Sometimes, she used the railway track behind the main street to pick up her brother, especially when she wanted to avoid the stares from this boy.

Grace finally met the boy, Alvin, when he came across the street and spoke with her. After that, he constantly communicated with Grace whenever he saw her. Alvin was kind, caring, and eager to know Grace better. She was aware of her obvious limps and had insecurities but also wanted to know more about Alvin. He made her laugh, which was a distraction from the doom she felt in her life.

That summer, she would graduate at age seventeen. Grace expected to stay home and rest. The rule of their house was a 6:00 p.m. curfew—she and her siblings must be inside by that time. They were restricted from even the verandah. After graduation, she decided all the rules would be unimportant because she would only have one year to live.

Once graduation was over, Grace began sneaking out of the house at night to talk with friends under the streetlights, spending hours there until early morning. In Grace's mind, her death at eighteen was inevitable. She wanted to live and try thing, things like alcohol, dancing, smoking, sexual activities, socializing, and other things teenagers do, having good and bad times with friends. They fought amongst themselves and had brawls. Alvin played music as a disc jockey. They went into other communities for concerts and dancehall activities.

No matter what Grace did, she was always and forever in severe agony from her wounds. Nothing helped. Distractions worked for a while, but alcohol made it worse, and dancing was detrimental. The church was no longer a priority. Healing still lingered in the back of her mind, and she considered that, with her imminent death, all her worries and troubles would be over in a year or so.

Grace enjoyed getting to know Alvin. She was out at night without her mother's knowledge. Rose became aware of her sneaking through the windows and locked all the windows to prevent Grace from getting back in.

Rose tried to keep her from roaming the streets at night, but nothing stopped Grace. She hid blankets and pillows outside so that, when she and her friends returned after daybreak, they could cozily wrap up and sleep on the veranda. Being disobedient, feisty, and rebellious went on for years.

Slowly and consistently, Grace's personality and characteristics changed. She became disconnected from life and living. Grace was so angry but disguised it behind masks. When the distraction of the nightlife was over, the pain returned, aching, growling, and annoying her like someone slowly picking cells away from her organs. It never went away. She realized that her anger was starting to affect her relationships and way of life. Her whole body felt the effect of the cells that were sickled.

Grace stopped tolerating the bullying and teasing in the communities. She defended herself physically. She had vengeance in her heart for anyone who thought she didn't deserve kindness. Rose had taught her to be kind, have self-confidence, and not let anyone bully her.

But Grace was angry with her mother and wished she'd never given birth to her—then she would not have existed. No existence meant no pain. Granted, Rose was Grace's role model, but the pain affected Grace's judgment toward Rose. Why not blame Rose for her wretched life? Grace started to disrespect her mother with foul language. Grace exploded with hurt, anger, unfulfilled desires, unacceptance, and shame. She screamed at Rose regularly in disagreements. Grace's words were damaging to Rose. She saw the hurt and pain in her mother's eyes, but Grace knew her fury must be channelled, or she would detonate like a ticking time bomb.

One of Grace's friends, Richard, realized that Grace was rude and hateful to her mother. Richard reprimanded Grace and encouraged her to apologize. He suggested that Grace take time to know Rose and resolve the dispute. Grace never apologized for anything, but she wanted to feel less furious, so she decided to apologize and learn about her mother's attitude and personality to reduce their conflicts.

As time went by, the relationship between Grace and her mother improved. She knew her mother did not trust her or take her apology seriously, but she was willing to prove her sincerity to Rose. Grace fought hard to compose herself and controlled her temper. She continuously practiced patience and stayed calm each time there was a possibility that an argument would start. The relationship improved between Rose and Grace. She was happy knowing she did not have to disrespect her mother but could find another source to control her frustration.

This was when Grace bought a machete. From then on, she had 1.5 feet of steel in her backpack to defend herself from evil community members. These spiteful people would purposely step on her wound, in jest for all to see. Grace then struck out with the steel. Many were wounded, and the police got involved. In each case, the police found that Grace was defending herself.

Community members sought to understand the root of Grace's fury. They tried to avoid her and encouraged their children not to interfere or antagonize Grace. One day, when Grace planned to cause bodily harm to one of her tormenters, she decided incarceration was the least of her troubles. She'd stand up to anyone and everyone, the way Dean had wanted her to when Doris slapped her in the face. As she walked toward the tyrant, her friend Mel came to her and inquired what was happening.

Grace explained what she was about to do. Mel tried to discourage Grace from causing harm. She grabbed the backpack from Grace and ran through the bushes. Grace was livid. She could not use her bare hands to defend herself because it would hurt. Grace did not attack the girl, and the incident went away.

Her brothers defended her, but Grace loved them and was afraid for them to be imprisoned. She was never the one to start a confrontation but would not back down or let anyone treat her like an undesirable. Community members began fearing Grace and she was left alone in her misery.

DOS AND DO NOTS

INFORMATION FOR PARENTS

1. Do not hurry your child but have patience with what they are going through.
2. Be there to support them without judgment or assumptions.
3. Assist them with resources to channel their anger.
4. Build trust so they can freely confide in you.
5. Take your child's problems and plight seriously because a troubled mindset can lead to severe mental illnesses.

INFORMATION FOR CHILDREN

1. School is a crucial stepping stone in learning who you are and what you want to become. Take advantage of every opportunity to find your natural talents and gifts so that you can use them to better your own life as well as the lives of others.

2. Learn all you can, when you can, and use the information to better yourself and the people around you.

3. If you do not have to stop attending school, do not stop. Whatever the circumstances, pull through.

4. Be proud of what you are doing. Remember, there will be those who are better than you and those worse than you. Do not compare yourself with others.

5. Always be yourself. Do not change a good characteristic because of peer pressure. Be the change agent for those who need to do better.

6. Some people will try to help you do your best. Appreciate them and let them know you appreciate them.

7. Despite the anguish you might be experiencing, find it in yourself to show gratitude and respect toward your parents, family members, or strangers.

AFTER GRADUATION

An important aspect of education is learning how to control the mind so we can free ourselves from mental troubles and distorted thought processes.

POSTGRADUATION, MORE COMMUNITY members tried to fix Grace's life. Jehovah's Witnesses endlessly stopped at the white picket gate and looked over to the veranda, wanting to convert Grace into their faith and practices. She listened out of respect. Some of these witnesses told her that God knew best, that God understood what she was going through, and that God was able to do unimaginable things. Then they repeated stories of God's plans for her life.

These words held Grace close to the edge of faith. People from her church told her stories about God, and she read some of those stories in the Bible for herself. She envisioned being one of those people in the Bible, experiencing change and harmony in her body so she could go out with her friends without being teased and laughed at. She imagined getting dressed without starting hours in advance to complete the task. She visualized wholeness. She felt and tasted a new life: a life without wound care, without slowness, without limping, without shame, and without tears and frustrations.

Grace would sit on the veranda, and her mind wandered into a futuristic time and space. She saw herself going to college and becoming successful in fashion design. She saw a runway with models modelling her designs and creations. She saw a free flow of movements, a pain-free life, and she heard laughter in her dreams and fantasies.

She was so desperate to live a life without fear. Grace would send messages to God with people who were old and were preparing to die. She told them to tell God that she needed the pain to stop. She needed healing, and it must come from him, no one else. Grace's heart held secret visions of criteria of what her life must be like, but doubts crept inside her soul and affected her clarity.

Alvin helped Grace with almost everything. He and Rose provided money for treatments. Grace did expensive ozone therapy for about a year, unsuccessfully. She soaked her legs in seawater. All it did was burn and cause severe discomfort. Alvin loved her and gave Grace everything he thought would make her happy. But the only thing that would make her happy was a pain-free life, even if that meant unhealed sores. She could live with the sores, but the pain was unbearable.

People brought different remedies for her to try: bushes, herbs, baths, and prayers. Grace got angry and told them that if God could use others to heal her, he should be able to heal her himself without their help.

DOS AND DO NOTS

INFORMATION FOR PARENTS

1. Celebrate with your child and be proud when they accomplish their graduation milestones.
2. Walk with your child to the next step in their journey.
3. Be a part of their story but not their narrator.

INFORMATION FOR CHILDREN

1. The world is at your fingertips! Reach for it and claim it.
2. Celebrate your graduation.
3. Rewrite your story.

HATER OF GOD

When hate consumes your entirety, there is no space or place left for freedom—there is only anguish, pain, and death.

GRACE WAS TIRED of the suffering and anxiety that gripped her every day. She saw the skies, stars, seas, trees, and unique things in creation. She felt the wind and was taught about the God of Jacob, Abraham, Daniel, Shadrach, Meshach, and Abednego— and all the miracles God performed.

She wished for a miracle. When miracle workers and great evangelists visited her town to preach and heal, she sat in the front row of their crusades. Her heart begged for a change. Healing would allow her great opportunities.

The numerous visits to the crusades and churches and listening to the Word of God stole her dreams and hopes. Everything she'd learned about God as a child became a distant memory. Grace's soul was no longer satisfied with the good things she used to believe about God—all her preconceptions crumbled in the face of her harsh reality. As her faith diminished, so did her will to live. She realized that the famous God who held the universe did not care for her.

In her soul, she knew God existed. There was no doubt in her mind that a powerful source held the universe in its hands. Grace decided that this God did not care enough about her needs. She decided that God kept people on strings like puppets, toying with their lives. He directed them where to go and what to do.

The more she thought, the clearer things started to become. She saw what no one else seemed to understand: that this great influencer had power. He did marvelous things but on his own time.

Grace realized she was not a part of God's plans. Her life did not indicate that God was loving and caring. She hated her life and refused to wake up to see the bright, shining sunshine. Every new day caused a piece of her to die. Her hatred grew toward God. She did not want to see a new day and the sunshine taunted her. Grace felt like God was mocking her hopeless future.

She continuously told herself that this life was hers, not God's. If he loved her, why was she in so much distress, despair, and despondency? Why would God allow an innocent girl to be so sick, with no resolution? Was it a family curse that needed to break? Grace decided to take control of her life because God did not own her. She wanted God to know that her control did not fall under his supremacy. Her destiny was in her hands, and there was nothing God could do to stop her. His power had nothing to do with Grace.

Grace was enraged when the Jehovah's Witnesses tried to speak. She shouted and told them not to return to her house. She did not want to hear about Jesus or God. The preaching of God drove her crazy. Nothing about those names gave Grace comfort.

She realized that, even with the new love with Alvin in the air and socialization on her terms, her spirit was restless. Her heart felt warmth when she was doing wrong and evil activities. She felt more comfortable retaliating. Her philosophy became "An eye for an eye," and "Do unto others what they do to you." She felt a sense of relief when others were repaid for their deeds.

She was tired of seeing the sunshine day in and day out. Every time the sun rose, the horror of being alive increased. The agitation allowed Grace to plan ways to escape this unfair and miserable world. She knew why she could not stay in this world, but the how, when, where, and what still needed to be worked out.

Grace regularly sat on the veranda and pondered what life would be like for her loved ones when she was not around. She knew her family would probably be relieved because she saw the sorrow in their eyes when they looked at her, especially when she cried. She believed that all would be well when she was gone.

Rose had faith and constantly, secretly prayed for healing for Grace. Grace saw the sorrows her mother carried and the hope she bore. Grace was twenty-two years old, and the doctors had been mistaken about her death. This made her resentful and suspicious of those in health care, except the senior specialist in the Sickle Cell Clinic. He was caring, and he never assumed what his patients were going through. He did a lot of research to provide the best care for his patients. This was comforting, so Grace decided to explore all options before committing to the end goal of walking among the dead.

Grace thoroughly thought it through. She visited the specialist and discussed health plans for maximizing adequate living conditions. She tried to eat well, but sometimes her discomfort disrupted her healthy meal plans.

It was difficult for Grace to sleep. When she fell asleep, it felt like worms and ants were crawling inside her wounds with twitching and stabbing sensations. The tingling and discomfort woke her up.

She could not continue her education. It took dedication and commitment to complete an uninterrupted course. Grace was unwell the day the examination was held for the Community College (CC) entrance. She did not get the opportunity to start CC like her counterparts.

Grace had no more game left in her soul. She had unhealthy relationships because her troubled heart needed to be fixed. She loved herself and had never conceived bad thoughts about herself but had no intention of living in such torment.

She was physically weak, limping around and stopping every few steps to ease the pain before completing her journey. Sometimes she wished she had someone to carry her to reduce the strain on her lower body. One side of Grace's body was longer than the other due to deformation and contracture in her right foot. Her muscles were underdeveloped due to a lack of exercise. She was unbalanced and often fell from tripping over her feet.

Grace's thoughts were beyond her young age. Her mind was uneasy with contradictions: wellness and illness, friends and foes, right and wrong, dying and living, love and hate, good and evil, belief and unbelief, and peace and restlessness.

Her immediate family supported her in both her healing journey or declining health. The world she knew despised her having to live with sores. The greenery and sunshine spoke of prosperity, but the disturbances in her soul highlighted failure. The only vocational pursuits she tried were fashion designing and fashion illustration. She was passionate about sewing and making new and unusual clothing, but it was not enough to quiet her questions about life and death.

Financially, she was stable. She was an entrepreneur because Rose and Alvin wanted her to have uninterrupted funding so she could stay home and relax. Grace's money was used for doctors, medications, grooming, clothing, socializing, and remedies. No matter what she had, her soul was empty. Life was unfulfilling, and death crept over her. She knew that living was not for her. She didn't belong in this world.

There was only one thing she desperately desired and that was painless wounds. Grace expressed this to the sickle cell specialist and told him that she wanted her legs to be amputated so she could better facilitate her own well-being.

This middle-aged man examined Grace in horror and could not believe what he heard. She supported her request by explaining how the different aspects of her life were not able to maintain her health. She told the practitioner that she could save her money and afford prostheses, which would serve her best.

The specialist realized the seriousness of the conversation and scrambled for words. He had not expected this discussion. He finally told her that she was too young to have her legs amputated.

Grace defended her treatment goal and told him she was old enough to make an informed decision. He told Grace he had seen ulcers healed; she was young and still had a chance. He was firm in his decision. Grace left the clinic feeling defeated.

Grace was heartbroken. Every time she did wound care, her wounds had unbelievable amounts of slough in them. There were no areas of healthy tissue. The specialist said there was nowhere to debride, but all Grace wanted was amputation. She would rather face life with prostheses than with unhealing sores. He kept telling her the wounds were not infected, but the pain said otherwise. The sickle cell specialist tried to give her hope, but Grace's heart was darkened with hatred for God, sadness from pain, and a desire to commit suicide.

Every day, Grace sat on the small rectangular-shaped veranda with whitewashed walls, a polished cherry-red floor, and fashionable built-in columns. She planned how and to whom to distribute her treasured possessions. Silently and secretively, she gave her things to her close friends.

No one knew what she was doing. She did not breathe a word to anyone. It took months of courageous and strategic mind games to outwit God. To beat God's evil mastermind and inconsiderate love.

Grace bravely prepared her heart for what was next. She was so strong, standing up to God and his foolish edicts. He hurt and taunted her daily with the bold, shiny sun that Grace wished she had never seen. The dazzling yellow brightness was everywhere. It peeped through windows, over the hills, and into the valleys, bathing everything in warmth. But Grace was unable to appreciate its purpose.

The sun's brilliance was a reminder to her that God, with his powerful designs and rhythmic cycles, didn't care about what Grace wanted or craved. He deliberately did everything to sustain a life that Grace did not want.

She wanted to choose a time, date, place, and conclusion that would make her extremely proud. Even the Maker of the universe would see how serious she was about her destiny. Grace was undeterred and took months of deliberate planning to get it right.

She had the perfect plan—something no one would expect and on a day when people would be at work. It was finally working out the way Grace wanted. What could go wrong? At last, Rose could be at peace and put her prayers for Grace's healing to rest. Rose was a dedicated Christian and expected greatness from God, but Grace knew better.

Every time Grace tried to tell Rose who God was, Rose silenced her and said she was speaking foolishly. Rose told Grace that she was ungodly and should stop talking nonsense. Rose looked at Grace with pity when she spoke about God in total disregard. She wondered if her daughter was losing her mind. Grace wanted to stay calm for the next few days. Soon it would end.

DOS AND DO NOTS

INFORMATION FOR PARENTS

1. Hate can be stamped on a person's spirit after continuous pain and discomfort. Monitor your child to ensure they are safe.
2. Monitor for suicidal ideation. Watch for red flags such as isolation and secretly giving away valuable items.
3. Encourage self-esteem and self-confidence so children feel love, acceptance, and belonging.
4. Monitor your child for subtle or significant changes in attitude and help them regroup.

INFORMATION FOR CHILDREN

1. Tell someone about your trauma. Give someone you trust the opportunity to assist you.

2. Do not isolate yourself because this opens you up to damaging thoughts.

3. It is hard to hold on to dreams and hopes but try it one day at a time.

4. Know that if something should happen to you, you would be missed by at least one person, so touch one life at a time.

5. Do not forget that you are loved and appreciated, even when it does not feel that way.

THE DAY BEFORE

With tunnel vision, each day resembles the last. A replica of the past influencing the present and leading to the end. There is nothing in between, nothing in the future.

THE SUNDAY BEFORE the finale, Grace walked to the Baptist church alone. Her heart laughed and her mind soared in contentment. She slowly walked and decided to converse with this big, mighty, great God who thought she was his puppet.

Grace told God that the day of her great event would be tomorrow, Monday morning. She told him the time, place, and plan. She said, "You are the only one I'm telling. No one knows except for you. It is out of respect for your existence that I want you to be aware." She continued, "You cannot do anything about this decision, and you cannot stop me from taking my life. It is my life, not yours," she said, feeling proud.

It was the first conversation she'd had with God in a long time. She explained all the things and feelings she had hidden from him and how she was relieved to be getting rid of him and herself once and for all. Grace felt that whatever happened after this day would be her choice, no one else's, and it was something she was willing to die for.

Grace entered the church from the side door. She walked with pride and a feeling of freedom and ownership. As she went through the door, the pastor stopped what he was doing and looked straight into Grace's eyes. He said, "Someone is planning to kill themselves tomorrow at Cornwall Regional Hospital at 10:00 a.m. by jumping from the tenth floor."

Grace stood in shock and astonishment. She said nothing, and the pastor held her gaze and repeated himself: "Someone is planning to take their life tomorrow at Cornwall Regional Hospital, 10:00 a.m., by jumping from the tenth floor." Grace was enraged. She had only told God about this a few minutes ago. Now God was trying to control her again, as if he were the boss.

God was trying to embarrass her in front of the congregation. The pastor continued pleading with Grace by repeating himself, saying that someone was planning to commit suicide tomorrow at Cornwall Regional Hospital at 10:00 a.m. by jumping from the tenth floor.

Standing behind the congregation, Grace wondered why God had told the pastor about the most important decision of her life. Indignantly, she spoke to God inwardly. "Do you think I care that you're revealing this information to the pastor?" Grace hissed. Grace hated God all the more and swore no one would own her life except her.

The pastor would not stop disclosing what God had told him. The congregation turned around to stare at the person the reverend was looking at. In Grace's heart, she knew she must go to the altar and surrender if she wanted the pastor to stop drawing attention to her. She held her head straight and saw the compassion in the pastor's eyes. He had known Grace since she was twelve years old.

Grace did not feel ashamed of wanting to commit suicide. She only felt rage because God had exposed her plans to the whole church. He had stolen her plans and tried to embarrass her in front of community members who would probably never forget that moment. The people stared at Grace where she stood. She knew she was just prolonging the drama, so she walked slowly toward the altar for redemption because the pastor was begging her to surrender her evil plan of wanting to commit suicide.

Grace went to the altar for a prayer of redemption, but she refused to ask for forgiveness because that was not her goal for the future. She hated God more and more as she stood listening to the pastor pray for her. Now she'd have to find a different way to end her life. Her mind was working overtime to accept the whispers and criticisms that were going on around her.

Some people had compassion and disbelief in their eyes. Rose was in church, but Grace could not decipher her reaction to the revelation. She received her prayers, and the pastor also requested that the congregation commit to keeping Grace in their prayers. She did not believe in prayer and was enraged to know that God had tried to prove himself superior in front of a crowd.

She vowed silently that this was not over. Grace felt like demons were directing her path and crawling through her mind. Ghosts of the past, present, and future surrounded her. Grace reasoned that, if she had not told God about her plan, he wouldn't have interfered. She went home troubled.

DOS AND DO NOTS

INFORMATION FOR PARENTS

1. Hang in there and continue to pray, if you believe in prayers.
2. Talk to your child and strategically explore their plans.

INFORMATION FOR CHILDREN

1. If you plan to harm yourself or others, do not do it. This should not be your last resort. You are worth much more.
2. The Creator sees and knows everything, even when things seem far-fetched.
3. Never underestimate the power of God in your life and the universe.

WHAT'S NEXT? THE VISITS

*Just because your mind forms a concept about something,
doesn't mean it is true. There are many dimensions to a concept,
and if you dig deep and are willing to explore,
you will find the answers.*

GRACE'S MIND WAS going haywire trying to find a different way to leave this earth. She fought for her well-being, especially when people whispered, gossiped, and did amusing stunts to disgrace her. Grace used words, stones, bottles, and anything else she could utilize as a weapon to protect her dignity.

There were a lot of feuds in the community regarding Grace's illness. Apart from the few friends who were dedicated to protecting her true character from backbiting gossip, her siblings were the only ones to protect her, especially Mick.

Grace had been unable to kill herself and now hoped that she would get severely hurt in one of the community brawls and die. The strife left people more afraid to mock Grace, and they walked on the other side of the street when they saw her.

She went to many crusades where people seemed to be healed, but the pastors had nothing for her, even when she sat in the front seat. All that spit fell on Grace from the men of God, yet she was still not whole.

People talked about Obeah/voodoo and spiritual healers. When Grace took buses and taxis to these people, she would always leave before seeing any of them. On one occasion, when Grace was leaving an Obeah woman's property, she ran after Grace and shouted, "I could see that you did not believe while you were coming up the hill." Grace walked away and left her.

Grace believed if God could use anyone to heal her, he could do it himself. One morning, Alvin came to Grace and told her that the Obeah man in the community wanted her at his shrine so he could heal her. Grace was livid. In her fury, she screamed at Alvin. She told him to tell the evil Obeah man that if he could heal her by cursing God, then God, who was more powerful, could do it himself. Grace told Alvin never to return with messages from the Obeah man again.

Grace was exhausted from lack of sleep because of the pain that crept through her body. Pain indirectly affected her eating habits. She was unbalanced. Migraines blinded her constantly, and she hid from the brightness of the world. Grace banged her head regularly on the wall, just wanting the headaches to go. If she shook her head, she could feel something moving inside her skull. It felt like she had displaced her brain within her skull. Her muscles were weak and her skin pale.

Demons visited Grace at night. They walked through the house and came to the bedroom window. Some sat or stood over her and watched. They tried to torment her. They held her down, lay on and beside her, and choked her. When Grace confronted them, they ran through the house and fled. They tried to plague her mind and whispered what they should do to her. She was not afraid of them. Her only fear was living in a world of pain that lingered from unhealing wounds.

Grace's spirit was less restless when Jesus came to visit at night. He would come to her when it was most quiet. He would have conversations but never spoke about her sores. On one of his visits, Jesus touched Grace's upper thigh with his right index finger and pointed over to Darlene's bed.

Grace turned and saw Darlene lying on top of her young baby. The baby was suffocating. Grace shouted Darlene's name, and she woke and tried to revive the baby who cried and gasped for air.

Grace returned her focus to Jesus to ask him about her wounds, but he was gone.

She lay there whispering to Jesus, "Why do you always come and ask me to help others, but you never stayed long enough to discuss my illness and my sores?" She continued, "This is frustrating and inconsiderate."

She never understood the significance of his visits. Jesus read her mind in conversation or indicated what he wanted. He would stay for a while and then leave when the conversations ended. At times, Grace did not get to talk about herself but would listen. She heard everything in the calmness and silence.

On the night of the baby's incident, Grace looked at Jesus for the first time. He stood at her bedside between the two beds. When he touched her, she turned her attention toward him. Grace saw Jesus before he pointed to her sister's bed.

He wore a whitish-cream robe. His skin was not white or black but olive-coloured. There was a glare and a shine that emanated from his black, shoulder-length hair. It shone like nothing she had ever seen, like soft, oiled wool. Grace looked directly into his face and saw kind brown eyes.

These visits were constant. They caused Grace to fall asleep after daybreak, which became her routine. Sometimes, she told her mother about these spirits. Her brother Dean laughed until the day he met them. Dean came to Grace and revealed that he knew she was speaking the truth after his encounter with these evil spirits. The fear of meeting them was in his voice. He thought it was because he'd stayed out too late and started coming home earlier. At least Rose and Dean knew and realized Grace was not losing her mind.

It was hard for people to believe the experiences and encounters Grace had during the night. Some friends thought she'd made them up; others were afraid to be with her at night. When she tried to prove these things to Alvin and Cathy, her best friends, they fell asleep before the spirits arrived. Grace did not know how to prove these things. And as much as she wanted to die, she did not want an evil spirit to kill her.

DOS AND DO NOTS

INFORMATION FOR PARENTS

1. Do not dismiss what your child tells you, even if it seems unbelievable. If you do, you will crush their confidence, and they'll think they are crazy.

INFORMATION FOR CHILDREN

1. You might have visions or encounters that seem weird, or hallucinations from your trauma and pain. Do not feel bad about them.
2. Always question what you are not sure about. Do research and get the facts before making decisions.
3. Miracles happen every day. There is a day for you, so keep believing.

WHY ME? WHY NOW?

A treat or a threat is awaiting the unbeliever if they desire to find God, or his opposition, the Devil. What shall you receive? Whom are you seeking? The Living God will show up when you least expect it—and so can his opposition.

GRACE'S MOTHER WAS relentless with them going to church. During the summer of 1999, the church advertised its crusade frequently. Rose was excited and went to the prayer meetings in preparation for the big event. The prayer team interceded for weeks before the crusade. The church members went to the community squares, pleading for people to commit their lives to God.

Grace wanted nothing to do with God. It irritated her just to hear the word *God*. She felt hurt and uncared for by this God. Rose expected her children to attend the crusade every evening for five evenings—and to be saved. Rose reminded Grace and her siblings about the crusade, but Grace did not intend to go anywhere near God or his words.

On the first night of the crusade, Rose obsessively reminded Grace that she was not leaving her behind. She waited for Grace to be ready, and they took a taxi to church together. The hatred Grace felt toward God was unexplainable.

Inside the church, members were getting things ready for the service. Community members were slowly filling the church. The praise and worship started. Grace was conflicted, silently cursing the people who were lifting the name of the Lord. The evil lioness in Grace roared against God's people. The more she loathed them, the more the people sang, clapped, and worshipped.

The internal ruckus caused Grace's mind to writhe in fury. Under her breath, she told God how much she despised him. She told him that he'd never cared for her and that the people who were worshipping were being fooled. They were oblivious to the fact that they were puppets God had on a string. He did not love anyone but just laughed at them.

The worship got louder, and people surrendered their all on the altar. Their eyes were closed. Hands lifted and voices roared. Grace's mind and body were plagued with resentment toward God. Internal voices told her to leave, but her mother would be unhappy if she did. Grace knew with her soul, body, and mind that God was powerful but evil.

There was the church pastor and the visiting preacher. They moved into the aisles and touched people who fell over in the Spirit. Grace thought the people and pastors were crazy. She knew they did not understand God the way she did. People spoke in the language of God, and God seemed to be responding to them. Some fell to the ground and were convulsing.

Grace sat on the wooden bench in the fifth row. The animosity built inside her body. She held her head down, hidden by the seat in front, and placed it in her hands. It seemed like an eternity. She willed the service to stop, but the pastors and congregation were on fire for God.

Someone touched her right shoulder. She looked up and saw the pastor of the church. He told her the preacher at the pulpit was calling her. Grace grew extremely indignant and told him to get away. She hung her head in her hands, cursing God again in her heart. There was another touch on the same shoulder. She looked, and the pastor indicated the preacher was calling for her. Grace told him no, go away.

Grace held her head in her hands again. As the so-called Spirit of God moved through the church, the pastor touched her right shoulder again. Grace did not know what happened, but she found herself running to the altar, uncontrollably screaming, "Hallelujah, praise God!" It felt like something had lifted her and flung her before the preacher.

She found herself worshipping God, the same God she hated. The visiting pastor told her, "God said tonight is your night. And you will never be the same."

He continued, "God said he has caught all your tears in his hands. He said you are healed from today forward. Starting today, you will never be the same." The pastor spoke in tongues intermittently.

The preacher continued as he looked at Grace. "He got all the messages you sent. 'You are lifted and will go places and speak of me,' said the Lord."

He told Grace things that God wanted her to know. She worshipped and did things she did not think were possible. Grace found herself dancing, singing, clapping, crying, and laughing. In a world where only she and God existed, she was calling out the name of Jesus in thanksgiving—in an act of total surrender and acknowledgment. Every shout caused her body to vibrate with uncontrolled jolts.

Grace was worshipping because of the things the preacher said no one knew. She knew God was in their midst because she felt different. Her body was pain-free, and she felt joy and peace that passed all understanding (Philippians 4:7). There was freedom. She felt like a bird in the wind, and Grace soared in the love of God. Nothing in the universe could have prepared her for that moment and her experience with God. It was surreal, and it was a feeling she wanted to get used to.

The congregation was on fire. They shouted, clapped, sang, danced, ran, fell on their knees, and lifted their hands. Grace did not remember if the pastor preached a sermon. She fell in love with God that day and wanted to stay in his presence. She didn't want to leave the church and was afraid it would be a dream.

Grace wondered why, at that moment, God decided to show up. Why, from amongst the whole congregation, had he decided it was her turn, her breakthrough, her healing, her redemption? Was it because she'd hit rock bottom? Was it because she was tearing him down to the ground? Did God want everyone to recognize that he was God and no one beside him (Isaiah 46:9)? He needed people to know that no one was outside or apart from him. He must show humans who he was, and no one could stop him. Everything was on his terms alone.

He showed up after fifteen long, lonely, desperate, disastrous years. God showed up. Grace knew she was going to die. She'd told herself over and over that the day she was healed would be the day she died. It was time for her to prepare her funeral, pick a burial spot, pay for a funeral service, and finally lie in peace,.

Grace was at the altar praising and worshipping this God she'd spent most of her life competing with. She was free and felt free at last. The night belonged to her and God. He had finally opened the gateway for her to enter. Grace had never experienced such joy, peace, or hope. There was no future like the one God gave.

The pastor told her that God had said, "Tonight is your night." He continued, "After tonight, you will never feel the same. Your tears I catch in my hands, and I count them all."

The pastor revealed, "You will go places and talk about me. I will lift you high and no one can put you down."

The preacher shouted under the direction of the Spirit, "You will speak of me and testify of things I did."

Grace felt a sense of totality and healing and knew everything would be okay. This love was what she had always searched for but felt unable to grasp. Grace was happy. She had longed for such a feeling.

At the end of the first night of the crusade, Grace felt intoxicated with love for God. She prayed constantly because she was certain it was the end of her life's journey. There were a lot of bad habits she needed to break.

Grace broke a record by going to services every night at the Baptist church. The praise and worship ended. People were healed, devils cast out, and the dead raised (Matthew 10:8). The visiting pastor went home. She was left alone to pick up the pieces without the fellowship of a congregation.

She lived in prayer and fasting to treasure what she had received. Grace kept asking God if her healing was real because she wanted to serve him.

It took approximately six weeks for Grace's ulcers to heal. She did not have to do wound care. She watched in amazement as the sores healed. Her nervousness settled, and she slept like a baby.

In Matthew 13, Jesus tells the story of a farmer sowing seeds in his field. The seed represents faith in him, and the soil is a picture of the human heart. Sometimes the seed falls along the hardened path where it cannot take root; other times, it falls on thorny or rocky soil; and sometimes, it falls onto good soil that's soft and ready to welcome it. When Grace surrendered her life to God, the seed of faith took root in her heart. Her life lay before her, and she would have choices to make. Would she return to her old ways or serve God in spirit and in truth? Her new journey had just begun.

DOS AND DO NOTS
INFORMATION FOR PARENTS

1. If your child does not believe in God, don't force them. Pray for them and provide facts so they can make informed decisions.
2. If they find God, do not discourage them but act as a support system.
3. If you do not believe in miracles, that is okay. Let others experience their miracles and talk about it.

INFORMATION FOR CHILDREN

1. If you experience a miracle, do not be afraid to talk about it. It might save someone else's life.
2. Your beliefs and values are important. Change on your terms.

INFORMATION TO HEALTHCARE PROFESSIONALS

1. Medical issues might disappear unexplainably. Have an open mind—not everything is medical. Some cases need spiritual intervention.
2. Do not discourage people from their beliefs.

REFERENCES

Laurier (website). 2025. "Seven dimensions of wellness." Laurier: Students. https://students.wlu.ca/wellness-and-recreation/health-and-wellness/wellness-education/dimensions.html.

Smith, Matt. 2024. "What Complications Can Sickle Cell Disease Cause?" WebMD. https://www.webmd.com/a-to-z-guides/sickle-cell-complications.

Tivoli, Ya, and Richard M. Rubenstein. 2009. "Pruritus." Journal of Clinical and Aesthetic Dermatology. National Library of Medicine. https://www.ncbi.nlm.nih.gov/pmc/articles/PMC2924137.

Trottier, Evelyne D., Samina Ali, Marie-Joëlle Doré-Bergeron, and Laurel Chauvin-Kimoff. 2022. "Best practice in pain assessment and management for children." Canadian Paediatric Society. Last modified February 20, 2025. https://cps.ca/en/documents/position/pain-assessment-and-management.